# The Puzzle of Autism:

# Putting It All Together

*A Guide to Transforming the*

*Treatment of Autism*

*For Parents and Physicians*

G.F. Gordon, MD, DO, MD(H) and

Amy Yasko, PhD, ND, NHD, AMD, HHP, FAAIM

Reprint – 2nd Edition

ISBN: 0-9759674
Matrix Development Publishing
Payson, Arizona

*This book is dedicated to Missie, Jessie, Cassie, Sloan, and Mark. Being blessed with healthy children is what inspires us to help others so that they may have the same pleasure in their lives.*

*A special word of thanks are owed to Edward Yasko, Alexandra Van Cleve, Christine Blake, Nancy Guyon, Elizabeth Horn Nelson, Christopher Higgins and everyone else who has assisted in the task of taking an individualized program and helping us to expand it into a generalized protocol.*

*We also thank all of the parents who have given us the opportunity to help their children to reach their full potential.*

# Contents

# Foreword

**Finding Dr. Amy**

It was a cold day in February 2003. My son Michael was looking at the snow on the runway as we approached Metropolitan Detroit airport. Michael, now 8 years old, was diagnosed with autism in 1997 at the age of 20 months. We were returning from one of our many trips to cities around the United States. The search for help for Michael had been continuous for four years. We had been working through one DAN (Defeat Autism Now) Protocol treatment after another in hope of recovering Michael. During this period, we consulted with many competent and caring doctors, yet I knew our treatment plan was incomplete. For the previous eighteen months, we had been focusing on toxic metal chelation, and were not making any real progress. The chelating agents kept wreaking havoc on his gastro-intestinal tract causing constant starting, then stopping to treat GI dysbiosis, and then starting up again. I was determined to find another way!

I started searching for alternative chelation approaches, and as fate would have it, I discovered Dr. Garry Gordon's website. After reading several pages, I noticed that Dr. Gordon kept referring to Dr. Amy Yasko, a researcher and practitioner from Maine. After reading and re-reading everything on Amy's website, I was excited. I started to feel energized with renewed hope. Had I found someone who could take Michael to the next level? Would his path to recovery now run through Maine? The next day I phoned the office only to learn that it would take six to eight months to get started! Amy was becoming well known around the country for treating autism and many other inflammatory neurological disorders. A long waiting list had developed.

**The Protocol**

Finally, in June 2003, I received a call from Amy's husband Ed. Amy was ready to get started with Michael. I was a little apprehensive about starting because we had just committed

Michael to a three-month stay in Atlanta. He was to begin a rigorous detoxification protocol at a well-known environmental medical clinic. I recalled how excited I was to discover Amy earlier in the year, and I was not going to miss out on this wonderful opportunity for Michael. We started both protocols simultaneously! I was very impressed by Amy's focus to detail in recording Michael's symptoms with me and in going over his files and files of lab results. Amy quickly customized a plan for Michael that was thorough, yet precise, and had a logical sequence to follow. The science behind her approach was convincing and the sequence just made good sense. The best part of all was that her plan for Michael was recovery. Anything less was unacceptable.

In reading this book, you will discover a great deal about the medical origin of your child's autism, how viruses and toxic metals result in excitotoxins causing devastation to the central nervous system, and how the brain can truly be healed after these toxins are removed. It is an intensive protocol that requires highly committed parents to be successful. I have found that combining Amy's protocol, with traditional laboratory testing and functional naturopathic monitoring, has worked very well for Michael. It has been extremely exciting and motivating to receive weekly lab results tracking excretion of toxic metals. Of equal importance, this protocol answers the tough question about what to do when the toxins have been removed and full recovery has not been achieved. For this difficult question, I am particularly grateful to Amy for step three entitled, "Program for Nerve Growth and Myelination". This is where Michael is now. It is truly joyous to see our son re-emerge without the dreaded backward slides that we were accustomed to seeing.

**Where We Are Today**
The protocol has evolved and expanded significantly over the past year through careful monitoring of each child's progress and through collaboration of Dr.Yasko with Dr. Gordon. We have made numerous adjustments in treatment intensity and type. Amy is

never content to merely achieve recovery.   She is constantly searching for ways to shorten the time frame.

As a result, Michael has made tremendous progress in recent months.  Although his recovery is not yet complete, we are seeing daily improvements, causing much excitement at home and at school.   For the first time, I can envision the complete and full return of our son from this horrific period in his and our lives.

I am confident that the protocol will continue to evolve, and rapidly. My advice to parents is to simply adopt this protocol and commit whatever is necessary to implement it.   Never lose sight of the ultimate goal.  Recovery!  From the experienced " tried everything parents" to those dealing with a recent diagnosis, this book delivers a "how to" approach that gets results.

*Robert Claeys*
Ontario, Canada
June 2004

X

# Preface

I feel privileged to participate in the development of this protocol for the full restoration of function for ALL autistic children - no matter how many other programs they may have already tried with varying degrees of success or failure. My colleague, Amy Yasko, with her background in molecular biology, immunology and infectious disease, is uniquely qualified to have developed a new perspective to this challenging disorder that continues to steal children away by the hundreds every single day.

My life's work has largely been centered around heavy metal detoxification. My website provides extensive documentation that everyone, child and adult, will have provable benefits by lowering their level of heavy metals through detoxification with oral chelation. Although I have been involved in trace mineral metabolism for over 35 years, there are always new developments that we must be aware of in dealing with today's proven levels of heavy metals and other pollutants that are now known to be adversely affecting the health of everyone on earth today. Some of these new developments are so powerful that they require a complete reevaluation of everything we thought we knew about the adverse effects of trace metals on our health. For example, we are faced with an epidemic of neurodegenerative diseases including Alzheimer's, ADD, ADHD, Multiple Sclerosis, ALS, etc. Heavy metals are clearly a major contributor to every one of these diseases. Autistic children are a case in point. After a lifetime of research in my field, my work with Dr. Amy Yasko has brought such radical new information to my attention that I am compelled (at age 69) to help re-educate the world, and help rewrite the textbooks on subjects like mercury and lead toxicity. This knowledge will help to bring effective therapies to the millions of patients around the world now afflicted with these neurodegenerative diseases.

Thanks to Dr. Yasko's work, we now have scientific validation that everything we thought we knew about heavy metals, and how to diagnose and treat these problems, was seriously deficient. She has patients where, according to the old rules, low levels of toxic metals in the urine after a provocative chelation challenge test should have indicated that further heavy metal detoxification for that patient would have been a complete waste of time and money. Dr. Yasko, with the help of dedicated parents, has found that negative urine-provoked tests for heavy metals may often mean nothing. She has demonstrated that RNA-based metal detoxification therapies can remove huge quantities of toxic metals from children who had received prior aggressive oral and/or parenteral chelation therapy with little or no benefit. The excellent results we are able to document have been achieved even after prolonged courses of DMSA or DMPS, frequently given by injection, had only marginal effects.

It is serendipity of the best kind that brought Dr. Yasko and I together at this point in our careers. We were both appointed to the board of NFAM (The National Foundation for Alternative Medicine) in Washington DC. We met at a dinner, and she started to tell me about the promising results she was getting in heavy metal detoxification using an oral EDTA based formula, the very product that I had formulated. When she began to tell me about the unbelievable increases in urine and fecal excretion of mercury, lead, antimony, cadmium etc. she was documenting using the Doctors Data Lab (whose work I have the greatest respect for), I had to learn more. She believed she was seeing these results because she had combined low doses of oral EDTA, Malic Acid and Garlic along with newly developed RNA products that when used properly are able to significantly lower the total body burden of pathogens. I knew then that we must work together.

Until that time, I was instructing all of the doctors doing chelation therapy that chelation therapy was only part of the treatment; getting the metals alone out was NOT enough, and in fact, effective chelation really requires a lifetime program because the earth is so polluted today. I had also emphasized the need to deal with the chronic levels of inflammation found today in virtually every chronic degenerative disease from cancer and heart disease to Alzheimer's disease. This inflammation has many contributors but it is due, in part, to chronic, low-grade infections in the body, which we now know that we all carry at all times throughout our life. Until I met and started to work with Dr. Yasko, my approach to dealing with both inflammation and pollution was so labor intensive, time consuming, and expensive that patients rarely adopted my comprehensive approach to achieving optimal health until cancer or another catastrophic disease was already present.

Dr. Yasko has one of the broadest views of anyone working in the field of autism. She understands that this disorder is a complicated puzzle and that full recovery requires an individualized approach - one that deals with each detail consistently over a prolonged timeframe. Dr. Yasko also understands that diet affects the activity of our genes and, as she has discovered, that nothing speaks as precisely to our genes as RNA, the molecule involved in cell-to-cell communication. Dr. Yasko is using RNA in this protocol to achieve levels of recovery in these children that may not have been possible otherwise.

However, I believe that the biggest use for RNA based research may not be as drugs, but as nutrients in new personalized nucleotide dietary supplement based programs using recently developed, unique, highly specific, extracted and purified nutritional products because of the information they can help convey.

The potential of RNA is validated by increased focus from a variety of areas within the scientific community. There are nearly 2000 new papers on RNA for medical indications published each year and over $2 billion has been spent worldwide by pharmaceutical companies trying to exploit the enormous potential of RNA. A recent article from Archives of Environmental Health, a publication for the National Institutes of Environmental Health, strongly states that research in RNA represents the most exciting development in biology of the decade, and that RNA research should lead to cures for cancer, AIDS, heart disease, ALS (amyotrophic lateral sclerosis), arthritis, etc.

In an article from the June 2004 issue of Discover, biochemist Jack Szostak hypothesizes that RNA based life may have existed before DNA based life and informs us "that the roles of the RNA in the cell have expanded beyond what any one imagined". RNA based therapies should be a key factor in helping develop the new paradigm of personalized medical practice to which the recently completed Human Genome Project must lead. Increased knowledge of our internal information network and the new gene expression microarray chips now being used in biomedical research will help us bypass the excessive current reliance on a pharmaceutical-based approach to medical care (see *Transducing the Genome* by Gary Zweiger). In fact, a new field of Bioinformatics is developing and information about millions of nucleotides is now stored in huge databases that the "new medicine" will be based on. It would appear that RNA's function might be as the "mother of all information networks."

This exciting new RNA technology will evolve into a convenient way to meet the need for preventive and health-promoting strategies for everyone, including safe and effective, documentable detoxification. Now we KNOW that autistic children, even those who are severely impaired, can completely recover. We are planning to develop a simplified version of this program for less severe problems (like ADD and ADHD, depression, OCD and other behavior or learning difficulties). Using this comprehensive RNA-based protocol for autism, a program that includes detoxification and lowering the pathogen burden, I see a way to improve the mental and physical health of every child. By supporting the body in every possible way, it is able to heal itself and lower its levels of various pathogens. When this occurs, the toxic metals that were locked inside cells are released in quantities never seen before in my years of working with trace minerals and chelation-centered heavy metal detoxification!

RNA based nutritional supplementation is the wave of the future, but we must recognize that giving RNA nutritional support without selecting what is appropriate for the particular needs of a patient will do some good and will clearly do no harm, but it is like playing all the 88 keys on the piano at the same time: you have sound but not music. I believe that the program we have put together for autism uses a variety of new specialized RNA based nucleotide dietary supplements to play the exact music these children need to hear in order to be well.

*Dr. Garry Gordon*
Payson, Arizona
July 7, 2004

XVI

# The Puzzle of Autism:

## Putting It All Together

*A Guide to Transforming the*

*Treatment of Autism*

*For Parents and Physicians*

# The Motivation

*"For years, Dr. Amy Yasko, an accomplished scholar, researcher, and clinician, has been quietly helping individuals recover from autism and other neurological disorders without drugs, injections, or other stressful, invasive procedures. As the parent of a child who has benefited greatly from Dr. Amy's expertise, I am delighted that Dr. Amy has written a book, which shares her blueprint for reversing autism with a wider audience. Parents and professionals seeking accessible, easy-to-implement, and most importantly, effective treatments for children or adults who are 'on the spectrum' will find this book to be an invaluable tool."*

Mary W. Hopkins, Ed.D.
Mother of Alex, age 18

Autism is reaching epidemic proportions in this country and the world. Parents are desperately looking for answers. Physicians who work in this field are overwhelmed and often unable to help the older or the most severe children. There is an overwhelming need for a comprehensive approach to autism.

We have developed a protocol that has made a significant difference for a number of children of all ages, and all severities of autism. Word has spread about the success of our approach. We realized that in order to help each person who has contacted us, we needed to find a way to move from individualized programs to a more general protocol. Rather than taking another year to work on this book and explain every facet of this problem exhaustively, we have focused on what parents and practitioners really want — an approach that will work for all the doctors and parents who need it now.

We don't have the luxury of fully explaining every issue here. We realize you will need supplemental information. Our goal is to share our knowledge and results with you. We urge you to look at the additional resources section of the book. It will direct you to websites with newsletters, chat rooms, audio and videotapes and other written literature. We have included a section of sample data to give you specific information from children who have used this protocol. This is to help you understand that this is not a theory; it is a program that we have used and are continuing to use. We are not suggesting that it is a magic bullet; quite the contrary. The detailed protocol described in this book is not a cure all and it is not a quick fix. It takes time and patience.

No book can replace the individual consultations we have, or the customized programs we design for each child. This protocol is designed to assist each practitioner in his or her practice. The idea is to share a proven protocol and provide a basic understanding of the pieces involved. Helping these children requires a comprehensive approach; one that takes into account all of the pieces, not just a single piece of the complex puzzle of autism.

We have made an effort to acknowledge some of those outstanding individuals who have brought many of these individual pieces to light. We apologize in advance for failing to mention all of the others who work relentlessly to help bring all of these children back to health.

# The Puzzle

*"Prior to having worked with Dr. Amy, I thought that it was up to me and me alone to get my son well; but how? This was perhaps one of the most daunting aspects regarding his illness. During the past several months we have seen great progress with Mitch. One of the most important things I've come to realize is I do not have to do it alone! I have found an inner peace knowing that Mitch is on the road to recovery. Together, Dr. Amy and I are working to get my child well."*

Margaret Wilson
Mother of Mitch, age 7

Sometimes a number of seemingly unrelated events occur simultaneously resulting in disaster. A prime example of this was the death of Princess Diana. If she had been wearing her seatbelt, if the car hadn't been speeding, if the driver hadn't been drinking, if the paparazzi weren't chasing the car...eliminate any one of those factors and a tragedy might have been averted. The multitude of factors that must occur to create the condition we call "autism" can be viewed in a similar fashion.

If an MTHFr mutation was not present, if there was less of a heavy metal burden, if there was no chronic viral infection, if no underlying streptococcal infection existed, if we didn't have excitotoxin damage, ...the negative cascade of neurological events that ends in a spectrum disorder may not have happened. So autism can be viewed as the puzzle, created from these various biochemical, genetic and physiological factors all careening together in the body of a developing child. To make informed decisions about undoing the damage that has been done in this "crash" of negative factors, each piece of this puzzle must be examined carefully, its function understood, and balance restored.

This book will look at each piece of this puzzle, as we understand it at this time, and suggest supplementation programs to address potential imbalances. The information presented reflects the most current view of the process of neurological inflammation that results in "autistic-like" behaviors, including the entire spectrum of autism-related diseases. This field is evolving almost daily with new information and new literature, and we will evolve with it. We expect that there will be additions, modifications and revisions to this book as new information comes to light.

There is not yet complete agreement between your authors on every detail in the proposed treatment plans (like all doctors, we are greatly influenced by what has worked for our patients). But the two of us bring well over sixty years of combined experience, and a passion for finding answers for what have seemed to be impossible problems (always utilizing the least toxic and most natural approaches) to the enormous challenge of autism. We will not give up until every child is given the chance to recover; until all of the pieces of the puzzle fit together, and this chronic disease no longer threatens the next generation.

This protocol cannot answer every question with regard to autism or other types of neurological inflammation. This is a starting point and we envision that individuals who are following this protocol will take advantage of the website www.autismanswer.com. This site will continue this initial effort, permitting questions and answers from health professionals learning to use this protocol, and another discussion group separately for parents working with this protocol. This protocol does, however, provide an explanation for many of the observed behaviors and symptoms that are associated with autism; a framework from which to help reverse many of these traits, and a rationale for why many of the currently utilized therapies are effective.

# Understanding the Individual Pieces

*"After 2 years of taking our son to Doctors around the US that address one area of the complicated biomedical puzzle called autism, we were fortunate enough to find Dr. Amy. Dr. Amy examined all the pieces of our son's chemistry, not just one. She didn't try to fit him into a shoe that didn't fit, but created one for him that did fit. Our very affected son made more progress in 2 months working with Dr. Amy than he had made in the last 2 years. He continues to improve before our eyes. Dr. Amy has given hope back to us. She has helped us to begin to reclaim our son and our life."*

Dave & Jennifer Larson
Parents to Cade, age 3 ½

In autistic individuals, imbalances have been shown to occur in a number of organ systems, neurotransmitters, and biochemical processes in the body. These include excess excitotoxins, heavy metal toxicity, methylation deficiencies, chronic viral and bacterial infections, fluctuations in serotonin, norepinephrine and dopamine, and liver, pancreas, stomach, intestinal, adrenal, thyroid and hormonal imbalances.

It is possible to rebalance all of these systems. This is true for any child with autism; there is no magic age or age limitation for this approach. However this is a process, it is a marathon, not a sprint. It takes time and patience. Success can be achieved by calmly correcting each imbalance. We liken this effort to the years of effort and expense some go through in restoring a classic car to its show room elegance. We are convinced that tremendous brainpower is present in autistic children and we are dedicated to helping them let it shine.

# Excitotoxins

Excitotoxins will continue to damage more nerves and wreak more havoc in the body if they are not addressed. Therefore the excitotoxin imbalance is the best place to start to put the pieces back together. Once excitotoxins are under control, it is easier to balance the rest of the body. This is an area where we encounter disagreement with some of our colleagues. The reason we are holding to our approach is that we have been able to help children who were not helped by approaches that ignored the vital role of excitotoxins in inflammation. Due to a basic lack of understanding about the involved chemistry, we find that glutamic acid, glutamine, etc. are still being included in supplement regimes for their potential gastro-intestinal benefits, while their documented potential for contributing to the proven neurotoxic effects are being ignored. Every decision needs to be based on potential benefits vs. potential risks.

Over seven years ago, Dr. Russell Blaylock described the pathway of excitotoxin damage and the role it plays in neurological damage brilliantly in his landmark book on excitotoxins. He spelled out specifically how and why MSG, hydrolyzed vegetable protein, aspartame and related compounds have been proven to cause death of neurons beyond any reasonable doubt. More recently, this concept of excitotoxin damage has been found to pertain to autism. Excitotoxins are neurotransmitters such as glutamate or aspartate that can excite the nerves to death when their levels are not regulated properly. Foods or supplements that contain excitotoxins include MSG (monosodium glutamate), glutamic acid, glutamine, NutraSweet, aspartate, aspartame, and cysteine. Mercury and aluminum can trigger glutamate release. Minimizing glutamate is a differentiating factor in our protocol and has helped many autistic children significantly. Since our goal is to help ALL patients we believe this extra aspect of neurological disease must be recognized if we are going to provide the maximum potential benefits to our children.

8

Glutamate is the main excitatory neurotransmitter in the body. It is essential for learning and for both short-term and long-term memory. It is also the precursor to the inhibitory neurotransmitter, GABA. GABA is a calming neurotransmitter, and is essential for speech. GABA neurons damp the propagation of sounds so that a distinction can be made between the onset of a sound and background noise. (GABA is often used to help restore speech in individuals who have suffered strokes.) Problems occur if the normal process of regulation of glutamate malfunctions and if toxic levels of this excitatory neurotransmitter build up in the synaptic junctions.

The balance between glutamate and GABA is like a seesaw. Under normal conditions, when the glutamate side gets too high, the GABA side of the seesaw will increase and decrease the glutamate. Under normal functioning conditions, excess levels of the excitotoxin glutamate will convert to GABA. There seems to be a "disconnect" in this process for autistic children so that the excitatory neurotransmission is high (stims) and the calming neurotransmission is low (lack of speech). When conditions occur that throw off this delicate balance, then high levels of glutamate can accumulate while the levels of GABA remain exceedingly low. This would create a situation that would require decreasing the glutamate levels, and increasing the GABA levels in order to restore balance. Chronic viral infection (there is increasing evidence that all of us suffer from one or more of these chronic infections throughout most of our lifetimes) may be related to this disconnect between glutamate and GABA.

Acute viral infection can lead to Type I diabetes. In Type I diabetes the body makes antibodies against the enzyme that converts glutamate to GABA, leading to a "disconnect" between glutamate and GABA regulation. It is tempting to speculate that if acute viral infection can cause this disconnect, it is possible that chronic viral infection can also lead to a similar disconnect between glutamate

9

and GABA regulation. One final note on this conversion from glutamate to GABA is that the enzyme that is responsible for the conversion, GAD (glutamic acid decarboxylase) uses vitamin B6 as a cofactor for its activity. The use of B6 for autism is a longstanding part of the DAN treatment, pioneered by Dr. Bernard Rimland. It is possible that B6 has been acting to aid in the conversion of glutamate to GABA in addition to its other roles in the body.

Once this disconnect has occurred, the brain requires sufficient levels of oxygen and energy to remove excess glutamate. However, glutamate release leads to the release of insulin, which results in decreased glucose levels. The amount of glucose in the brain regulates the removal of excess glutamate from the synapses. Therefore, a drop in blood glucose disrupts this removal process and allows the build up of toxic glutamate. In fact, conditions of hypoglycemia, or low calorie/starvation conditions induce the release of glutamate and reduce the ability to remove excess levels of glutamate from the brain. This excess glutamate depletes glutathione. Glutathione is one of the most powerful antioxidants found in the body and helps to protect neurons from damage. Glutathione depletion consequently leads to the death of additional neurons.

Glutamate has six different types of receptors to which it can bind in the brain. One of these receptors, the NMDA receptor, is tied to calcium transport as its mode of action. In the case of the NMDA receptors, the release of excess glutamate triggers an inflammatory cascade that results in the death of neurons by the major influx of calcium into the nerve until it results in neural cell death. Normal levels of calcium result in normal neuron functioning. However, excessive levels of calcium make it impossible for the neuron to rest; the neuron continues to fire without stopping, causing the release of inflammatory mediators, the release of more glutamate, thus resulting in more calcium influx. The high intracellular levels of calcium also lead to high levels of nitric oxide and peroxynitrite, causing damage to the energy producing apparatus of the cells.

Magnesium (a second part of Dr. Rimland's protocol) is able to modulate the calcium flow, as is zinc. However, zinc is a double-edged sword as it is also able to activate glutamate release via the non-NMDA glutamate receptors.

Although these receptors are called "glutamate receptors", any of the excitatory amino acids are able to bind to the receptors and cause excitotoxin damage. The toxic potential of these excitatory amino acids has been suggested to be proportional to their ability to excite neurons. These excitatory amino acids include glutamate, aspartate and to a lesser extent, cysteine and homocysteine.

Glutamate and aspartate are common as food additives as well as naturally occurring components of a large number of foods. In cells, glutamate and aspartate can be synthesized from each other. In the presence of ATP, glutamine will convert to glutamate. The two main food additives that are sources for excitotoxins are MSG (monosodium glutamate) and aspartame (NutraSweet). High levels of glutamate and aspartate are found naturally in protein rich foods, including very high levels in wheat gluten, and milk casein. The process of making protein into a protein powder releases glutamate from its bound form, resulting in the ingestion of free unbound glutamate. While these amino acids are necessary for normal brain function, excess amounts of them create a wide range of bodily damage. Body systems that have been affected by glutamate toxicity include effects on white blood cells (elevations in the levels of eosinophils), effects on blood vessels (causing migraines and reduced regulation of blood pressure), and inhibition of the conversion of glutamate to GABA. Excess glutamate can cause vestibular dysfunction resulting in nystagmus. The sites in the brain that have been reported to be damaged by excitotoxins include the hypothalamus, the hippocampal neurons, and the Purkinje neurons, among others.

The recent finding that copper suppresses GABA ties together disruptions in copper/zinc ratios in the body to glutamate and GABA imbalances, which is yet another piece of the puzzle. These disruptions in zinc/copper ratios have been well characterized by Dr. William Walsh of the Pfeiffer Clinic. (Yet another piece of this complex puzzle comes into play, the successful use of EDTA as a standard in the supplement program of autistic children. EDTA will help to decrease copper levels. This will release the GABA from copper suppression, and will help to rebalance the zinc/copper ratio).

There has been a suggestion of a relationship between heavy metal toxicity and glutamate in the literature. As referenced in Aschner et al "In the absence of glutamate, neurons are unaffected by acute exposure to mercury, suggesting that neuronal dysfunction is secondary to disturbances in astrocytes." And "Co-application of nontoxic concentrations of methylmercury and glutamate leads to the typical appearance of neuronal lesions associated with excitotoxic stimulation." (Methylmercury alters glutamate transport in astrocytes. Neurochem Int. 2000; 37:199) this would suggest that lower concentrations of mercury might be more toxic in the presence of excess glutamate or other excitotoxins.

Excess levels of glutamate have been implicated in a range of neurodegenerative diseases, including Alzheimer's disease, Parkinson's disease, Huntington's chorea, stroke, Multiple sclerosis, and ALS. In the case of autism, irregularities related to glutamate have been observed. In addition, glutamate, glutamic acid and aspartate and aspartic acid were found to be elevated in individuals exhibiting autistic behavior relative to controls.

Children with autistic type behavior have often been described as exceedingly intelligent, even to the extreme point of being considered savants in particular areas. Dr. Tsien and his collaborators have demonstrated a correlation between glutamate receptors and superior ability in learning and memory. By overproducing a component of one of the glutamate receptors, they were able to increase the level of glutamate binding.  This was the first demonstration of a relationship between increased glutamate/ glutamate receptors and higher intelligence.  The down side of the enhanced level of glutamate was an increased risk of stroke and seizure activity.  This work suggests a potential correlation between intelligence and glutamate levels.  It also points to the potential increased susceptibility to excitotoxin damage due to excess glutamate/glutamate receptor activity as a consequence of enhanced intelligence.

While there have been reports that the density of AMPA-type glutamate receptors is decreased in autism, this may be due to receptor recycling as a function of glutamate binding rather than an actual lack of receptors.  Cells are constantly in the process of selecting and recycling receptors.  Recycling occurs, and is more complex in neurons.  In neurons recycling is complicated by the fact that internalized proteins have the possibility of returning to their surface of origin or to a second plasma membrane domain.  This would seem likely in this case, for although the receptor density was decreased, the mRNA levels of glutamate AMPA receptors were significantly increased in autism.

Regardless of the reasons for the glutamate excess in autism, it is a critical first step to remove excitotoxin triggers from the diet.  This involves reading labels and closely monitoring food and supplement intake to avoid excitotoxins.  The Appendix of this book contains a list of excitotoxins and the other names by which they are known.

## The Liver

The liver is one of the most important organs in terms of maintaining health.  It is the site for carbohydrate, fat and protein metabolism, storage of vitamins and minerals, and regulatory mechanisms for blood sugar and hormone levels.  Bile production, which is necessary for elimination reactions, also takes place in the liver.  In addition, and perhaps most importantly, the liver is the site for detoxification of the body. A central problem in the treatment of autism is the function and health of the liver. If the liver is healthy, it can make sufficient enzymes for the efficient detoxification of the body.

The liver contains high levels of enzymes that are required for detoxification processes. It contains one of the highest levels of glutathione, one of the most powerful antioxidants found in the body. Glutathione is essential for both the Phase I and Phase II detoxification systems of the liver. Phenol-sulphotransferase (PST) is another sulfur-containing enzyme that detoxifies leftover hormones and toxic molecules, as well as food dyes and chemicals. Metallothionein are sulfur-containing proteins that scavenge free radical and regulate metals. In the case of autistic children, almost 100% have low PST enzyme levels. Both the PST enzymatic detoxification systems, as well as glutathione require sulfur. The metallothioneins, MT proteins that are involved in heavy metal detoxification in the body, are also sulfur-containing proteins. This lack of sulfur seems to be a central problem with children exhibiting autistic behavior.

High extra-cellular levels of the excitotoxin glutamate cause the extrusion of intracellular cysteine resulting in glutathione depletion. Low levels of magnesium also result in decreased levels of glutathione, as does infection or inflammation that causes elevations in TNF alpha. Heavy metal toxicity may be exacerbated due to the lack of sulfur/glutathione detoxification systems; this heavy metal toxicity then triggers further excitotoxin release, which creates a continuous cycle of inflammation and depletion of antioxidants and detoxification proteins.

The function and health of the liver and pancreas appear to be at the center of many of the health issues seen in these children. While sulfur-containing supplements are useful as chelating agents, they are also serving to supply sulfur for glutathione, the PST enzyme system, for taurine, and as antioxidants.

## The Stomach, Pancreas, and Intestinal Tract

In an ideal situation, following the digestion of food in the stomach by hydrochloric acid, the HCL is dumped into the small intestine stimulating the release of several proteins. These proteins include gastric inhibitory peptide (GIP), secretin, and cholecystokinin (CCK). GIP slows the release of acid into the intestinal tract, secretin stimulates the pancreas to release bicarbonate to neutralize the acid, and CCK stimulates the gall bladder to release the bile (made by the liver) into the intestines to neutralize the acid and help digest fats. In addition, GABA release may help to reduce the triggering of transient lower esophageal relaxations, decreasing gastroesophageal reflux (GERD). GABA is also essential for proper intestinal motility. If, however, the pancreas and the liver are in a weakened state, this ideal situation will not occur. Instead, the HCL is still dumped into the small intestine, but these three proteins will not be released properly. This results in a situation where the intestinal tract becomes more acidic due to lack of released bile, and results in an environment that is more conducive to growth of microorganisms. The resulting microorganisms in the intestinal tract may contain a wide variety of anaerobic bacteria, including a number of species of *Clostridium.* In addition, there will be an overgrowth of yeast, *Eschericia coli*, and *Streptococcus*, rather than normal intestinal flora.

James Russell, a professor in the Section of Microbiology at Cornell University, Senior Research Microbiologist of the USDA, and a recognized expert in *E.coli* has stated that, *"Escherichia coli* is a common bacterium in the GI tract, but it is usually outnumbered by other types. *E. coli* is never a beneficial bacterium, but under normal circumstances the animal and *E. coli* tolerate each other. Some strains of *E. coli*, however, are not people-friendly, and these highly virulent forms can cause acute illness or even death."

In addition to creating imbalances in intestinal flora, an added result of insufficient bile relative to acid will be inadequate digestion of fats, consequently a decrease in absorption of fat-soluble nutrients (i.e. vitamins A, D, and K); and a sub-optimal amount of secretin and CCK to trigger communication with the brain. Decreased levels of CCK in the brain are correlated with anxiety and panic.

Secretin has been shown to potentiate the levels of CCK induced enzymes, and this may be an additional benefit associated with its use. Similar to CCK, the hormone secretin is found in the brain as well as the GI tract. Secretin has been shown to cross the blood/brain barrier. It is postulated that secretin that crosses over into the brain as well as secretin that is released by Purkinje cells in the brain may regulate cells nearby to produce GABA.

Neuropeptide Y is another peptide that is abundant in both the brain and the GI tract. In the brain it is involved in regulation of appetite, anxiety and blood pressure. In the GI tract Neuropeptide Y is involved in the regulation of pancreatic secretions and gut motility. Neuropeptide Y has been reported to suppress glutamate and antagonize the effects of glutamate.

Glucagon-like peptide is another gut peptide that is involved in associative and spatial learning and memory, and also involved in neuro protection from glutamate-induced damage.

Gluten and casein free diets have been found to be helpful in autistic children. Wheat, casein, and hydrolyzed yeast are concentrated sources of glutamate. Wheat gluten is 43% glutamate and milk casein is 23% glutamate. Consequently, a diet that is high in casein, gluten, and yeast would exacerbate a system that is already overwhelmed with excess excitotoxins. However, the milk protein casein and whey are powerful stimulators of CCK. Diets deficient in casein and whey could lead to further imbalances in CCK levels in the GI tract, necessitating additional stimuli for CCK.

On a related note, endocannabinoid synthesis is triggered in the brain as a protective response to excitotoxin damage. This protective release of endogenous cannabinoids could lead to elevated levels of opioids. These endocannabinoids in the brain also suppress the release of both CCK and GABA, further decreasing their levels.

The role of the pancreas in the conversion of glutamate to GABA has already been discussed. The pancreas is a critical piece of the autism puzzle. If the pancreas is not healthy the result can be high glutamate levels, low GABA levels, decreased secretin, decreased CCK, and decreased Vitamin K, among other imbalances.

## Vitamin K Deficiency

Excess stomach acid and insufficient bile (due to decreased liver function) creates a situation of relative acid excess and acid pH in the intestinal tract. (Ingestion of glutamate as MSG itself has been reported to cause excess acid and heartburn.) This would create an environment that is conducive to yeast, *E.coli*, and *streptococcal* overgrowth and non-ideal for normal protective bacterial flora. This imbalance in normal flora can be further exacerbated by the excitotoxin glutamate. Excess glutamate has been shown to increase the survival of enterohemorrhagic *E.coli*, particularly under acidic conditions.

While Vitamin K is a fat-soluble vitamin, it is not stored like the other fat-soluble vitamins; consequently it needs to be absorbed on a daily basis. Normally this occurs when the bacteria in the GI tract process leafy greens. If however, the normal flora of the GI tract has been disturbed there will be a Vitamin K deficiency. Most likely all children are born deficient in Vitamin K, as it does not cross the placenta.

Vitamin K is essential for healthy calcium metabolism, and has functions related to blood clotting. It prevents excessive bruising and bleeding; is important for strong bone and teeth health; and for sugar regulation (controlling hypoglycemic-related anxiety attacks).

It has also been shown that Vitamin K2 can help prevent pathologic accumulations of calcium in tissue, which we will learn is one of the critical factors leading to cell death. One of the highest levels of vitamin K in the body is in the pancreas, which is critical for sugar regulation in the body. Most children suffering from autistic behavior seem to have imbalances in their ability to tolerate sugars. In addition to the brain, the other area of the body that is able to concentrate the excitotoxin glutamate is the pancreas, which would result in further damage to the pancreas and sugar regulation.

Vitamin K reacts enzymatically with glutamate and calcium to ensure proper placement of the calcium in bones and teeth. In addition, Vitamin K is a cofactor for the conversion of glutamate to gamma carboxyglutamate. Lack of vitamin K would then create a cycle of deregulation in the glutamate/calcium pathway leading to further neurological inflammation.

## Streptococcal Infection

Dr. Vojdani, Dr. Bock and their colleagues have demonstrated the presence of antibodies to Streptococcal M protein, as well as autoantibodies against neuron-specific antigens in blood samples taken from autistic children. Under certain conditions, antibodies targeted against the basal ganglia of the brain have been found to follow *streptococcal* infection. *Streptococcal* infection has been implicated in leaky gut syndrome, as well as a wide variety of behavioral disturbances given the acronym PANDAS (Pediatric Autoimmune Neuropsychiatric Disorders Associated with Streptococcal infections) that have been described by Dr. Susan Swedo. In addition, Dr. Maddie Hornig and Dr. Ian Lipkin and their colleagues (Hoffman et al) have developed an animal model of *streptococcal* infection that results in motor and behavioral disturbances.

*Streptococcal* infection is known to lead to elevated levels of the inflammatory cytokines NFKB and TNF alpha. High levels of TNF alpha have been implicated in Tourettes syndrome, facial tics, obsessive-compulsive behavior, and schizophrenia. In addition, the level of TNF alpha is inversely correlated with glutathione levels. Consequently, high TNF alpha levels as a result of *streptococcal* infection would result in decreases in glutathione levels.

Generally, bacteria elicit a B cell mediated immune response, and viruses elicit a T cell mediated immune response. However, *streptococci,* all of which have the ability to nonspecifically stimulate T cells, elaborate a large number of extra-cellular toxins. Therefore, once an immune response is mounted against *streptococcus* it would involve both T cell and B cells resulting in a major inflammatory reaction. A chronic *streptococcal* infection could therefore lead to a depletion of both T and B cell mediated immune factors. Conversely, an inadequate T and/or B cell response to *streptococci* could result in chronic underlying *streptococcal* infection.

*Streptococci* are also known to elicit a number of other factors in addition to these toxins. These factors include streptokinase (which increases the inflammatory mediators TNF alpha and IL6), neuraminidase (which can aid in the establishment of viral infections), and NADase (which depletes NAD that is necessary for recycling of glutathione), and glutathione peroxidase (necessary for virulence).

Chronic *streptococcal* infections (i.e. ear infections) and the use of easily abused antibiotics (as noted in the book *The Killers Within: The Deadly Rise of Drug Resistant Bacteria)* that follows can result in a lack of re-population of the intestines with normal flora with a subsequent loss of Vitamin K. Consequently, the net results of *streptococcal* infection are depletion of Vitamin K levels, decreased glutathione levels, potential over-stimulation followed by depletion of the immune system, increased TNF alpha levels (which trigger OCD, facial tics, etc.), potential autoimmune responses and inflammatory reactions against various areas of the body including the heart, the basal ganglia and the GAGs in the GI tract.

*Streptococcus* may permanently reside as part of the bacteria or flora in the nasopharyngeal cavity of children who are highly susceptible to *streptococci*. The mucous system in our nasal passages flushes bacteria and viruses into our stomach. It is easy to see how under "compromised conditions", *streptococci* could survive the stomach and make its way to the intestinal tract. Gastric reflux has been implicated as a factor in ear infections. (Gastric reflux may be associated with low levels of GABA.) It is not surprising then to note that in addition to its role in ear infections and strep throat, *streptococcus* has been implicated in leaky gut. Gut flora changes play a major role in causing the increased intestinal membrane permeability that is seen with leaky gut. Depletion of glutathione is a common occurrence in leaky gut. *Streptococcal* infection, or the presence of chronic or recent infection, depletes glutathione levels. High glutamate levels also result in the depletion of glutathione. *Streptococcal* infection is also more likely to be an issue in individuals with high glutamate levels, as glutamate is related to virulence in *streptococci*. *Streptococcus* flourishes in a high glutamate, low glutathione environment. Thus, the combined effects of changes in gut flora and depleted glutathione lay the groundwork for leaky gut.

We know that if a child eats the same foods too frequently, the leaky gut will lead to that child's reacting badly to even the few foods that manage to survive the "do not eat list" that they seemed to tolerate well initially. With all these limitations, when we finally find something that our child likes, the danger is that we rely on it excessively. Until we have healed the intestine, the body can become sensitized to almost any food eaten too frequently. We recognize that there has to be some individualization to each child's diet as we pay attention to the research linking our blood type to foods that we should avoid as described by Dr. Peter D'Adamo. Furthermore, using food allergy testing to IgG and or IgE will generally find some foods to which your child has some acquired sensitivities. However, there is currently no test available in the United States that identifies accurately which foods are directly increasing the inflammation that is a major contributor to the entire autism picture, helping to cause the leaky gut as well as adding to the inflammatory process surrounding the nerves. New work by Dr. Ian Stokes describes a technique that analyzes the neutrophil response in blood incubated with reconstituted food samples. Using this process it is possible to detect foods that produce a neutrophil response and to construct a diet that avoids them.

## MTHFr Allelic Variation (MTHFr Mutation)

MTHFr (methylenetetrahydrofolate reductase) is an enzyme involved in folate metabolism. Certain genetically inherited forms of this enzyme do not function with optimal efficiency. As a result of this decreased activity, there is a shortage of methyl groups in the body for a variety of important functions. Methyl groups are "CH3" groups that are moved around in the body to turn on or off genes. The particular site of the MTHFr mutation creates a situation where the body is unable to form 5-methyl tetrahydrofolate (5 methyl THF) from folate. Supplementation with folate will not bypass this mutation. However, it is possible to supplement with 5 methyl THF, which will bypass the mutation.

Methylation is related to neurotransmitter levels. Methylation of intermediates in tryptophan metabolism can affect the levels of serotonin. Intermediates of the methylation pathway are also shared with the pathway involved in dopamine synthesis. Consequently, imbalances or supplementation of the methylation pathway will also affect the neurotransmitter dopamine. In addition to its direct role as a neurotransmitter, dopamine is involved in methylating phospholipids in the cell membranes, and has been extensively described by Dr. Richard Deth. This methylation of phospholipids helps to keep the cell membranes fluid. Membrane fluidity is important for a variety of reasons including proper signaling of the immune system as well as protecting nerves from damage. The role of membrane fluidity in nerve damage has been described in ALS and Alzheimer's disease.

Increases in certain inflammatory mediators, such as IL6 and TNF alpha, lead to decreases in methylation. Chronic inflammation would therefore exacerbate an existing genetic condition of undermethylation. The inability to progress normally through the methylation pathway, as a result of this MTHFr mutation, could lead to a build up of precursors of the methylation pathway, including the excitotoxin glutamate.

This altered MTHFR activity can lead to low levels of DNA and RNA synthesis, as the building blocks for DNA and RNA require the methylation pathway. This makes it difficult for the body to synthesize new cells. This would result in a decreased level of new T cell synthesis. *De novo* T cell synthesis is necessary to respond to viral infection, as well as for other aspects of the proper functioning of the immune system. T cells are necessary for antibody producing cells in the body (B cells) as both T helpers and T suppressors to appropriately regulate the antibody response.

In addition, the decreased level of methylation can result in improper DNA regulation. DNA methylation is necessary to prevent the expression of viral genes that have been inserted into the body's DNA. Loss of methylation can lead to the expression of inserted viral genes.

Proper levels of methylation are also directly related to the body's ability to both myelinate nerves and to "prune" nerves. Myelin is a sheath that wraps around the neuronal wiring to insulate and facilitate faster transmission of electrical potentials. Without adequate methylation, the nerves cannot myelinate in the first place or cannot remyelinate after insults such as viral infection or heavy metal toxicity. A secondary effect of a lack of methylation, hence decreased myelination, is inadequate "pruning" of nerves. Pruning helps to prevent excessive wiring, or unused neural connections, and reduces the synaptic density. Without adequate pruning the brain cell connections are misdirected and proliferate into dense, bunched thickets. Recent findings (Nature Neuroscience, Vol 7 April 2004) suggest that proper myelination is necessary to ensure the subsequent pruning of nerves.

Inadequate myelination and pruning of nerves as a result of decreased methylation may relate to the published MRI results of Dr. Martha Herbert. She has reported that the outer area of white matter in the brain was larger in autistic children than in controls, while the inner zones of white matter were not different. According to Dr. Herbert, the outer zone that showed the increase in volume is the area that myelinates later; this may help to elucidate a timeline for problems in myelination and pruning.

## Heavy Metals

The toxic effects of heavy metals, including mercury, have been well characterized and documented by Dr. Amy Holmes and Dr. Stephanie Cave among others. The heavy metal burden of our children is now being openly acknowledged by the EPA in their statements that over 600,000 babies are born each year with elevated levels of mercury. The sources of this mercury are ubiquitous since we release over 600 tons of mercury into the air annually just from burning coal for our electric power. Although autistic children do NOT usually reveal significant levels in their hair (since they appear to have a defect in their ability to detoxify mercury), they, like everyone on the planet, carry far higher levels of all toxic heavy metals than any humans did as recently as 400 years ago. Lead also averages 1000 times higher concentration in all human bones tested anywhere are earth today than four centuries ago. Levels of lead, mercury and cadmium are all found to be in far greater concentrations than what is recommended for optimal health and longevity. These heavy metals are contributing to the epidemic of degenerative disease we are seeing today in every country in all age groups.

Toxic metals accumulate in our bodies over our lifetimes beginning with the amounts we receive from our mothers during pregnancy, metals we are inoculated with during vaccination, and the metals we consume and breath every day thereafter. Dr. David Steinman and Dr. Samuel Epstein have written a comprehensive guide to the toxins in our daily lives that add to this total body toxic burden.

Many of the symptoms seen in autism resemble aspects of heavy metal toxicity. A number of treatment protocols for autism include metal chelation and detoxification and have proven successful in helping to reverse symptoms of autism. We have chosen not to use intravenous chelation agents whenever possible, rather to focus primarily on the use of oral and topically administered EDTA as our primary heavy metal chelator.

An important part of the protocol presented in this book includes a proprietary approach to metal detoxification that allows us to target metals that may be sequestered by virus in the body. We discovered that none of the available chelators eliminate these "bound" metals, so we developed a unique, oral, RNA-based process to aid the body in dealing with these chronic infections. We are pleased with the success that this new approach is providing and see clinical improvements along with significant increases in urine and/or fecal excretion of toxic metals. These results suggest to us that these chronic infections have been efficiently binding toxic metals in the body where no chelating agent seems to be able to effectively remove them. We have seen these results even with patients who have undergone extensive parenterally administered DMPS, to the point that others had been convinced that mercury was no longer an issue. Even in these previously treated patients, we are finding substantial releases of mercury as the viral load is being reduced. With this elimination of virus and heavy metals, we have also seen patients' symptoms improve dramatically.

It has been assumed that thimerosal (the mercury-containing preservative used in many vaccines) breaks down into ethylmercury in the body, and the released ethylmercury causes the toxicity problems. There is not sufficient evidence at this time to prove that this degradation process goes to absolute completion. One possible explanation for the tight association between virus and metals that we have observed is that some portion of the thimerosal may not breakdown completely to ethylmercury. Any intact thimerosal may mimic the actual building blocks for DNA or RNA synthesis. These "thimerosal building blocks" would contain the mercury molecule potentially creating a condition where the mercury is stably integrated into the nucleic acids, DNA or RNA. The lack of adequate nucleic acid building blocks due to the MTHFr mutation may be an extra inducement for the body to use unnatural building blocks. The mercurated nucleotides could be incorporated into the body's DNA or RNA, or into the DNA or RNA of viruses in the body. If this occurs, one would expect a situation where mercury is stably bound within the body and difficult to remove.

As an alternative to their potential incorporation into DNA and RNA, these mercurated nucleic acid bases could also interact and inactivate various enzymes in the body. Serving as "nucleotide mimics", mercurated nucleotides have the ability to interact with the TS (thymidylate synthetase) enzyme, or with the HGPRT (hypoxanthine guanine phosphoribosyl transferase) enzyme. Alternatively, once the ethyl mercury group has been cleaved from thimerosal, the remaining mercaptobenzoate molecule may be able to interact with and inhibit thymidinc kinase or thymidine synthase. If this were the case then one would expect that there would be additional imbalances in methylation and purine metabolism. If mercurated nucleotides interact with TK (thymidine kinase), it would have the potential to harm the host (the human body) without harming the virus. (A number of herpes viruses have been shown to lack a TK gene and are therefore resistant to the effects on the TK enzyme – conditions under which the human body would be susceptible.)

A third mechanism by which chronic viral infection may lead to the observed retention of heavy metals involves host metallothionein proteins. Viruses have been shown to induce the synthesis of host metallothionein proteins (MT). MT proteins help to detoxify heavy metals including mercury, and to balance zinc and copper in the body. It is documented that viral infection can cause an increase in the level of MT proteins that is directed by the virus. MT proteins that are triggered in response to viral infection are able to bind the heavy metals in the body. However, unlike MT proteins that are made in response to cellular signals, these viral-triggered MT may act to sequester the metals inside the cell. It is important to remember that viruses are parasites; they are not free-living organisms. It is in the best interest of the virus to keep "the host" (in this case the child) immuno-compromised so that the virus continues to have a home. If the virus were able to aid in trapping heavy metals inside the cells, it would certainly help to keep the host immuno-compromised. This later association of MT proteins, virus and heavy metals might also help to explain the lack of available host MT proteins in autistic children described by Dr. Bill Walsh. If viral infection has commandeered host MT synthesis, it would result in the observed decrease in host MT levels. If any one of the scenarios described above were occurring, it would help to explain the difficulty in removing heavy metals from autistic children. It would be necessary to eliminate chronic virus in order to fully eradicate heavy metals from the body.

There are a number of agents that are currently utilized for chelation of heavy metals including DMSA, DMPS, EDTA, glutathione, alpha lipoic acid, and garlic. Each of these agents has antiviral capabilities. Garlic is well known as an antiviral, antifungal, antibacterial nutritional supplement. Glutathione is one of the body's most important defense mechanisms against viruses. There are examples in the literature of EDTA eliciting virus from cells. DMSA, which is widely held as solely a mercury chelator, has been described to have antiviral activity; more specifically anti-retroviral activity (measles and mumps are retroviruses). DMSA is commonly used to help to chelate heavy metals and for detoxification with children exhibiting autistic behavior. However, it is important to realize that DMSA has been shown to trigger the inflammatory mediator TNF alpha so it would be important to use caution and to actively add agents that effectively can reduce and/or control inflammation when using DMSA. (We have been able to accomplish this anti-inflammatory effect consistently and conveniently in all of our patients with an RNA-based oral liquid product that is easily added to the treatment program of all children, since it can even be added to their food.) DMPS is also listed on the NIAID therapeutics database as showing antiviral activity against HIV. Both DMSA and DMPS have potential side effects and should be used with caution and under the care of a doctor familiar with chelation protocols.

It is possible that all of these chelating agents act to both chelate heavy metals as well as to trigger chronic virus containing metals from the body. The "detox rash" that most parents of autistic children are familiar with, may actually be in part a viral rash, as chronic virus is eliminated from the body.

## RNA Viruses

The positive rationale behind vaccination is to prevent more serious disease from active, acute, naturally-acquired infections. Natural acute measles, mumps and rubella infections have been known to have potentially serious repercussions including brain damage, deafness, and blindness and photosensitivity, in addition to neurotoxicity.

The particular combination of viruses used in the MMR vaccine is unique in that all three are single-stranded RNA viruses. Measles and mumps are negative-stranded RNA retroviruses, and rubella is a positive-stranded RNA virus. Human cells do not contain enzymes for copying their own RNA. As a result, the viruses bring in their own enzymes with them in order to initiate replication once they have infected a cell. The virus diverts the host's (the human cells) resources for replication of more viruses. One of the key components used by the virus for replication is the nucleic acid bases that are needed to produce more viral RNA. Once viral replication begins using the enzyme that the virus has brought in with it, along with host resources, many copies of the viral RNA are made. Required viral proteins are then made; the virus is assembled and packaged.

During this process the virus inhibits host cell functions. This serves the dual purpose of allowing the virus to commandeer the host machinery for its own purposes as well as to ensure that the host cell will die and release all the newly formed viral particles. The newly released viral particles are then free to infect additional cells. What happens if the viral particles are not released? The virus remains intracellular rather than completing the normal viral life cycle, and the result would be a chronic viral infection inside host cells.

It may be that the lack of normal flora in the gut, as well as already elevated levels of the inflammatory mediator TNF, an MTHFr mutation, heavy metal toxicity, and depletion of glutathione due to streptococcal infection set up a predisposing condition for problems with certain vaccines leading to a chronic viral infection. To further exacerbate the condition, it has been found that the tetanus toxin (from the DPT vaccine) can cause the lining of the intestinal tract to peel, leading to diarrhea as well as creating a lack of normal flora. In addition, tetanus toxin inhibits the release of GABA as a result of its action on synaptobrevin. (Vaccines are made by treating the toxins with heat or chemicals, such as formalin, which should denature the toxins). The subsequent vaccination of children with these predisposing conditions, with a live virus such as the MMR vaccine, may allow an otherwise attenuated and non- virulent strain to create an infectious situation by populating the gut. The gut would normally be protected by normal flora and sulfated NAC-glu molecules so that this would not occur. However, given the predisposing conditions, one could end up with the chronic measles infection that has been described by Dr. Andrew Wakefield, and the gut problems addressed by Dr. Jeffrey Bradstreet and Dr. Jerry Kartzinel. In addition to the measles infection, we believe that there are potential problems with chronic viral infections from each of the other viruses in the MMR -- mumps and rubella.

Retroviruses like measles or mumps also have the ability to copy their viral RNA into DNA. This DNA copy of the viral RNA is then stably inserted into the host DNA. As already mentioned, rubella differs from the other two vaccine viruses in that it is a positive stranded RNA virus. However, in the presence of retroviruses, variants of the rubella virus have occurred such that the RNA genome of the virus can also be converted into DNA. This DNA can then stably integrate into the DNA of the host cell, analogous to the situation for mumps and measles. The viral genes will be expressed unless the body has adequate methylation to prevent the expression of these inserted viral genes. Due to an underlying MTHFr mutation, in addition to the other puzzle pieces already discussed, it is unlikely that the body can prevent this chronic viral expression.

In the case of the MMR vaccine, one of the justifications for vaccination has come from the suggestion of associations between viral infection and diabetes. In the case of rubella virus, it has already been shown to be associated with diabetes. Babies infected with the rubella virus in their mother's womb, who are born with congenitally acquired rubella syndrome, often develop Type I diabetes. One study concluded that rubella virus can infect pancreatic islet cells and that the infection can severely reduce levels of secreted insulin. Like rubella, mumps disease has been strongly associated with the development of Type 1 diabetes. Similar to rubella virus, the mumps virus can infect pancreatic islet cells. It has been found that 85% of children with Type I diabetes have antibodies against the enzyme that converts glutamic acid into GABA (the GAD enzyme, or glutamic acid decarboxylase). This would result in elevated levels of glutamate and reduced levels of GABA. If the pancreas is not functioning optimally (lack of vitamin K, and too much glutamate in the pancreas) then the inflammatory mediators will become glycosylated (have sugars linked onto them), which then calls in more inflammatory mediators to the site. Therefore, many of the potential effects of acute viral infection appear to be similar to the observed issues seen in autism, and may be a result of chronic viral infection with measles, mumps and rubella.

In addition to vaccine issues associated with potential chronic viral infection, there is the issue of the preservatives themselves that are used to maintain the stability of injected substances. The preservatives can contain free glutamate as gelatin, which would directly trigger excitotoxin damage. Many children receive the chickenpox vaccine at the same time as their MMR vaccine. Varivax is stabilized with MSG. The Rotavirus vaccine (used approximately 8/98 to 10/99, 1.5 million doses) contained a contraindication for use specifically for individuals with hypersensitivity to MSG. Other preservatives include thimerosal, phenol, and aluminum. In the case of aluminum, it has been shown that the entry of aluminum into the brain is enhanced when it is coupled to glutamate. Aluminum, once in the brain, is able to trigger additional excitotoxin release and damage. As previously mentioned, mercury is also able to exacerbate excitotoxin damage.

## Herpes Viruses

DNA based viruses like chicken pox (Varicella-zoster, or herpes zoster) or Human Herpes Virus 6 (HHV6) can cause problems in addition to the potential problems caused by chronic infection with measles, mumps, and rubella viruses. Dr. Michael Goldberg, Dr. Jeff Galpin and Dr. Kendall Stewart have described the involvement of herpes in conjunction with autism, among others. HHV6 has also been implicated in the demyelinating disease of multiple sclerosis. Recently, HHV6 has been found to be directly correlated with seizure activity. Chicken pox is known to cause neurological damage, particularly during pregnancy. Similar to the situation with the MMR, the virus that is used for the Chicken Pox vaccine is a live attenuated virus. It may be that in individuals with the predisposing conditions already discussed, this virus is also able to establish a chronic infection. If this is the case, then cells that harbor the DNA of the varicella zoster virus may also lead to an accumulation of heavy metals. Other herpes viruses, such as HHV6, may be able to establish chronic viral infections in susceptible individuals with similar results. The potential role of herpes, and other DNA based viruses in autism, is an area that is still evolving.

## Other Chronic Viral Infections

A number of other viruses have been implicated in neurological inflammation including CMV (cytomegalovirus), EBV (Epstein-Barr virus), and RSV respiratory syncytial virus). It is impossible at this time to rule out a role for other chronic viral infections in autism. If virus contributes to the pathology of autism by virtue of helping to exacerbate heavy metal retention, then it is possible that any viral infection can be involved. Dr. John Martin of the Center for Complex Infectious Diseases (www.ccid.org) has made us aware of the existence of simian virus 40 (SV40) in early polio vaccines. This is seen in an article in the July issue of New Scientist that reports Soviet oral polio vaccines from the late 1960s found in a freezer at the National Institute for Biological Standards and Controls in the UK were infected with SV40.

Dr. Martin has also conducted additional work with atypical viral infections and believes that they too may be involved in autism. These atypical viruses have been given the name "stealth viruses" as they are able to evade the immune system and lead to chronic infection. These "stealth viruses" appear to have recombined with other genes of cellular, viral or bacterial origin.

Research by Dr. Jean Francois Bach may help to tie together viral infection with yet another piece of the puzzle. Normal individuals harbor autoreactive Tcells that do not attack organs expressing the corresponding autoantigen. For instance, T cells that are specific for myelin basic protein (MBP) or glutamic acid decarboxylase (GAD) can be derived from the peripheral blood of healthy individuals. The research from this group demonstrates that for an autoimmune response to develop, it is not sufficient for T cells to be specific for an autoantigen. The autoreactive cells must also, in addition, be activated. Viral infection has been reported by this group to be sufficient to activate autoreactive T cells.

## MHC/HLA Antigens

The MHC (major histocompatibility complex) is a group of genes that code for cell-surface antigens and are the principle determinants of tissue type and transplant compatibility. The HLA antigens are proteins on the surface of human cells that help to identify these cells to the immune system. Differences in HLA antigens are genetically determined.

Dr. Hildreth and his colleagues at Johns Hopkins (Gould et al) believe that the immune response to MHC antigens actually represents the body's original way of defending against retroviruses. They theorize that in the case of HIV, newly formed viruses should bear the HLA proteins from the people they are infecting at the time. If the virus then moves into a second person with dissimilar HLAs, the second person should mount an immune response to the virus.

Several of the live viruses used in vaccines are produced in either human female diploid cells (WI38) or human male diploid cells (MRC5). As the virus is grown and buds through the host cell membrane it picks up host cell components as described above. These components will include HLA antigens or sex specific surface antigens. Individuals with different HLA types may have varying immune responses to these injected HLA antigens as part of the live virus vaccine. Differences in antigenic responses to sex specific cell surface antigens may also be involved in immune responses. Looking at the HLA type of the cell lines used to make live virus vaccines might be worthwhile with an eye toward prescreening for susceptibility to autism.

Differences in susceptibility to measles vaccination have been found to be influenced by the HLA type of an individual. Similarly, HLA antigenic differences are noted for celiac disease, diabetes as well as a number of other autoimmune and inflammatory conditions. Dr. Maddie Hornig has presented results from an animal model that indicate MHC antigens play a role in determining thimerosal related neurotoxicity. HLA type is another area that will likely continue to show a role in autism in the future. It may be that individuals of particular HLA types are more susceptible to predisposing factors involved in this complex condition, similar to the male prevalence in autism that has been noted in the past.

## COMT Allelic Variation

As is the case for MTHFr, the COMT enzyme (catechol-O-methyltransferase) has several genetic variants. COMT is also involved in methylation. It is responsible for inactivating several of the neurotransmitters (dopamine, norepinephrine) through the process of transferring methyl groups. The different variant forms of COMT have differing levels of enzyme activity. Individuals with the low activity form of the enzyme would have higher levels of dopamine. Individuals with the high activity enzyme would be more likely to have lower levels of dopamine. In this complex puzzle of autism, dopamine is involved in methylation, therefore the levels of dopamine as a result of the COMT enzyme activity would reflect back on the MTHFr mutation and the methylation pathway.

COMT is also responsible for the inactivation of norepinephrine. Differences in norepinephrine and acetylcholine levels may be reflected in terms of the response to new situations. Dr. Yu and Dr. Dayan report that high levels of acetylcholine are associated with the ability to deal with expected uncertainty, while high levels of norepinephrine are required for unexpected uncertainty, as when the aspects of a task are unpredictably changed. Consequently, variations in norepinephrine levels may be a factor in the requirement for "sameness" by so many autistic children. The different allelic variations in COMT activity have also been associated with differential sensitivity to pain; the high activity form of the enzyme was related to better tolerance to pain. The low activity form of the enzyme resulted in greater pain sensitivity. The high activity form of COMT has also been implicated in schizophrenia. Conversely, the low activity form of the enzyme has been associated with rapid cycling bipolar disorder.

Estrogen may help to decrease COMT activity. The antioxidant quercetin is a good substrate for COMT and may also reduce its activity. The exact relationship between the COMT "mutations" and autism is still under investigation. It may be that the different forms of COMT are related to autistic children who are over, or under-methylators. The use of the "blink test" (average number of blinks/minute is between 15-30) may be helpful in the regulation of dopamine. The blink rate varies with the amount of dopamine; less dopamine means fewer blinks.

## Muscarinic Receptors/Acetylcholine

Acetylcholine is a neurotransmitter that acts on two types of receptors, nicotinic and muscarinic receptors. Nicotinic receptors are involved with sympathetic nervous system stimulation, while muscarinic receptors are involved with parasympathetic stimulation. The balance between these receptor activities is involved in the sympathetic and parasympathetic imbalances that have been noted in autism. There have been mixed reports when it comes to supplementation of choline to enhance acetylcholine levels in autistic children. Some children appear to respond quite well to

34

choline, while others have negative reactions. Choline supplementation can be particularly dangerous in children with seizures, as choline and acetylcholine have been reported to increase seizure activity. Some children have subclinical seizure activity that has yet to be diagnosed or treated; it can be especially difficult to make the correct judgment with respect to choline supplementation in this specific group of children. (To add to the complexity, vagus stimulation decreases seizure activity in drug resistant epilepsy; vagus nerve stimulation should cause the release of acetylcholine.)

It is important to consider all of the components of any supplement that you give to your children, as they may contain hidden sources of choline or other ingredients that may be a problem. Many transdermal delivery systems (topical delivery gels) contain lecithin as part of the delivery matrix. Lecithin is a source for choline. In addition soy lecithin in topical gel preparations may be a problem for individuals who are allergic to soy.

"Supplementary lecithin requires a special note of caution. Many people take lecithin either under a physician's guidance or from the vitamin counter to eliminate fats and cholesterol from the body. Lecithin is a natural substance that occurs in some plants and animal tissues and in egg yolks. One of its components, choline, is suspect for people with seizures. In a 1983 study, a choline-supplemented diet significantly increased seizures. The researchers concluded, "Our results suggest that supplementation of dietary choline above NORMAL levels might result in increased susceptibility to epileptic seizures. This could result from either a reduced threshold for seizure or from an increase in the rate of seizure development." This conclusion definitely suggests supplementary lecithin with its choline component is not the treatment of choice for people with seizures. (Taken from Epilepsy: A New Approach by Adrienne Richard and Joel Reiter, M.D., Walker and Company, New York, 1995)"

Excess levels of acetylcholine are regulated by the enzyme acetylcholinesterase, which causes the breakdown of acetylcholine. Although it is counter intuitive, a lack of acetylcholinesterase will result in a down-regulation of muscarinic receptors. Potentially this would have the unexpected outcome of <u>high</u> levels of acetylcholine, however with <u>low</u> levels of muscarinic (parasympathetic) receptors. It has been assumed that there is a lack of choline in autism. However, it may instead be a lack of acetylcholine muscarinic receptors. Muscarinic receptors are implicated in processing of cognitive functions, memory, problem solving, regulating pancreatic secretions as well as depressing glutamate release in both the prefrontal cortex and the temporal lobe.

A number of parents believe that their children began the "downward" slide following one or more of the DPT (diphtheria tetanus pertussis) vaccinations. As already mentioned, tetanus toxin (by its action on synaptobrevin) blocks the release of GABA and glycine. In addition tetanus toxin can also inhibit the release of norepinephrine, enkephalins, acetylcholinesterase, and acetylcholine. Tetanus toxin affects the hypothalamus, decreases hormone levels (such as testosterone), causes excessive sympathetic discharge with urinary excretion of catecholamines (i.e.dopamine) and can cause chronic seizure activity. Antibodies against the GAD enzyme (the enzymes that converts glutamate to GABA) have been reported in some cases of tetanus toxicity. Tetanus toxin binds irreversibly. Nerve function can only be returned by the growth of new terminals and synapses.

Toxoid vaccines are made by treating the toxins with heat or chemicals, such as formalin or formaldehyde. The rationale behind this inactivation process is that it <u>should</u> destroy the majority of the toxins ability to inhibit and affect neurotransmitters. However, the toxoid should still be able to stimulate the immune system to produce protective antibodies. Once these protective antibodies are made and bind to the toxin, it should eliminate the toxins ability to bind to the receptors on the host cell membrane. If the body is having difficulties with the immune system, it may be unable to mount a proper antibody response to the injected toxoid. In the absence of antibodies this may allow the toxoid to be free to bind to its target and to interrupt the release of neurotransmittors such as gaba, and glycine and to affect the level of acetylcholinesterase. This would have the consequence of creating imbalances in acetylcholine regulation, with the ultimate result of a decreased number of muscarinic receptors.

The quality control of toxoid vaccines is based on immunogencity and safety testing in animals, who are capable of mounting an appropriate immune response. This leaves open the possibility that the toxoid may behave differently in individuals who do not mount an appropriate immune response. Tetanus toxin behaves like a normal antigen in terms of the immune system, and as such it is recognized in a MHC dependent fashion. The carboxy terminal portion of the toxin is both necessary and sufficient for the ability of the toxin to bind. What this means is that if the carboxy terminus of the toxoid has not been sufficiently denatured it will still be able to bind synaptobrevin and have toxic effects.

> *In vitro* (test tube) analysis of binding activity found that:
>> "When *toxoid* or crude toxin is used, non-specific *cleavage of synaptobrevin* substrate occurs" (Kegal et al Federal Agency for Sera and Vaccines Germany).

This indicates that the vaccine toxoid can have similar effects to the toxin itself, especially in the absence of an adequate immune response. Therefore, tetanus toxoid may also be able to inhibit neurotransmitter release. Currently *in vitro* (test tube) tests are not used to monitor the efficiency of toxin inactivation by formaldehyde before use in vaccine preparations.

Nystatin has been shown to prevent cleavage of synaptobrevin by tetanus toxin. Nystatin has also been reported to induce liposome fusion, which may in part compensate for a lack of synaptobrevin.

Dr. Sidney Baker and others have described the role of yeast infections in autistic children. Nystatin is often used to treat these infections. Many parents comment on the finding that their children do better on nystatin even in the absence of a yeast infection. It is possible that in addition to its action as an antifungal, the nystatin may be acting to aid in the release of neurotransmittors that have been compromised by tetanus toxoid.

Just as there are "over methylators" and "under methylators" with respect to the methylation pathway, there may be children with different levels of acetylcholine or acetylcholine receptors that in part are determined by their reaction to the DPT vaccines. There may also be a genetic component to this complex piece of the puzzle. We have observed that there is an association between autism and the presence of family members with asthma. The condition of asthma itself is associated with elevations in acetylcholine as well as viral infection (the viruses most commonly associated the asthma attacks are RNA viruses). The microcosm of acetylcholine regulation itself is beginning to emerge as its own complex puzzle within the larger puzzle of autism.

We have had preliminary success in utilizing supplements to enhance muscarinic receptor activity; use of acetyl-L-carnitine, MSM, ashwagandha and ginkgo may be helpful for this purpose. The use of nystatin may also be helpful. In addition, the amino acid alanine has been reported to reverse the inhibitory effects of phenylalanine on acetylcholinesterase activity. It is not known if the use of alanine would help to reverse effects of toxoid inactivation of acetylcholinesterase activity, if that is indeed occurring.

This area is still evolving and is not fully resolved at this time. However, it is important to consider imbalances and irregularities in this system in any treatment plan.

# Putting the Pieces Back Together

*"The most beneficial changes I have seen in the least amount of time, in both my sons, is using Dr. Amy's program. These are significant changes socially, verbally, and emotionally. And believe me, we have done just about everything!*

*Knowing exactly what supplements to give, how much and what each will do is such a big relief after doing this on my own for so long. I wish I knew about Dr. Amy when each of my children were first diagnosed.*

*More metals are coming out now than with the DAN protocol. Getting rid of virus and supporting the immune system are such big keys in the autism puzzle.*

*Tailoring children's treatments according to their symptoms and behaviors makes a big difference. Dr. Amy understands what is going on, not just with the child, but with the family as a whole."*

Erin Griffin
Mother of Kyle age 8, and Brendan age 11

## General Considerations

"Autism Spectrum Disorder" is a catchall phrase, and children with very different biochemical imbalances are put together in this category. Therefore, while there are some universal generalities, the specific plan of treatment depends on the individual needs of each child. However, there are some guidelines that apply to any neurological supplementation program. First, it is recommended that you <u>work in conjunction with a healthcare practitioner</u> when utilizing a detoxification program. Working with someone who has experience in detoxification will be helpful even if they have not used this particular program before. They will have a good idea of what to expect during detoxification and how to deal with the physical and behavioral changes you might encounter through this process.

The program should begin with a really good general supplement that covers the vitamins and minerals, and is high in antioxidant supplements that will lay the groundwork for the more specialized supplements. Preferably this supplement will not contain iron, as iron can exacerbate neurological inflammation. Iron is also necessary for virulence of many bacteria, including streptococci, so limiting iron is useful in limiting bacterial infection, which could trigger additional inflammation. Kyolic garlic has been shown to be effective against ear infections and may be useful in dealing with Streptococci. Also, because of the inherent problem with zinc/copper ratios in many autistic children, any general supplement you choose should not contain copper. Oxidative stress can have pleotropic effects on the body and on inflammation, as has been described by Dr. Woody McGinnis and others specifically with respect to autism. Consequently, the use of additional individual antioxidants in conjunction with a strong antioxidant general vitamin will help to address the issue of oxidative stress.

A hair mineral test, urine test (available from Doctor's Data in Illinois) or a blood test can be used to ascertain that there is no deficiency of copper since prolonged administration of zinc in the absence of copper theoretically could lead to a potential of copper deficiency. In addition, calcium should be included only in limited amounts, and should always be balanced by magnesium.

Individuals should get more sulfur/glutathione into the system in as many healthy ways as possible. Glutathione can be well absorbed transdermally and sublingually. There are also a number of sources that have specially formulated glutathione for oral delivery. Glutathione is also delivered via an IV push as well as through the use of a nebulizer. Caution should be used with these later two forms of delivery. We are personally aware of several children who have shown sensitivity to glutathione. Systemic administration, or administration directly to the lungs can be extremely dangerous if a child has an anaphylactic reaction to glutathione. Reduced glutathione is reportedly the more potent form of glutathione; NADH can be used as a supplement to help recycle reduced glutathione. The use of NADH is especially important for those using glutathione via an IV push. If NADH is not supplemented then the body may "steal" NADH from other internal pathways in an attempt to recycle the glutathione. We have seen cases where children became depleted in NADH after the use of IV glutathione without supplementation with NADH. In these cases the Krebs cycle may become compromised.

There are also a number of supplements that will indirectly boost glutathione levels, these include: milk thistle, alpha lipoic acid, N-acetyl-cysteine/vitamin C, MSM, aloe and rosemary among others. While glutamate (or glutamic acid or glutamine) and cysteine are precursors in the formation of glutathione, they are also excitotoxins and will trigger more inflammation in the brain; therefore it is best not to use those items directly as supplements to boost glutathione levels. Foods/supplements that are naturally high in sulfur include garlic, broccoli, onions, and foods high in quercetin.

If the liver is healthy it can make sufficient glutathione -- one of the most important antioxidants in the body. The liver is also critical as the site of detoxification of waste products for the body. Anything that makes the liver healthier will help; this would include some of the supplements already mentioned such as milk thistle, carnitine, NAC, dandelion (also high in vitamin A), as well as SAMe and B vitamins. The use of depakane (valproic acid) can deplete carnitine. Children who are taking valproic acid to reduce seizure activity should consider supplementation with carnitine.

In individuals where chronic yeast or fungal infection is evident, it is important to restore the normal functioning of the intestinal tract.

*Chloride blocks sulfur*

*NADH keeps GSH reduced*

Supplement with a really good source of vitamin K, agents to limit yeast formation (which occurs as a result of lack of normal flora) and digestive enzymes. Supplements that will help with digestion and yeast overgrowth include lactoferrin, digestive enzymes, and probiotics.

Individuals should consider supplements to help to detoxify the excess glutamate in the system. These would include branched chain amino acids (mixture of leucine, isoleucine and valine only), pycnogenol, and grape seed extract. Magnesium is critical as it regulates the excess calcium from flowing into the nerves and killing them. Epsom salt baths (magnesium sulfate) are useful particularly if the bathing water is high in chloride and fluoride. Chloride blocks the action of sulfur in the body. Limited amounts of zinc and calcium are fine, but too much will increase nerve damage.

Supplements that add energy (oxygen and ATP) to the brain will help it to detoxify the inflammatory reactions caused by excess glutamate and heavy metals, which trigger glutamate release. These supplements include ginkgo, vinpocetine, NADH, CoQ10, ribose, and carnitine. It is important to use NADH with glutathione to maintain the glutathione in a reduced state. Carnitine actually helps to increase the energy in the mitochondria, which are the energy producing organelles inside each cell. Carnitine is also useful in repairing liver damage. Acetyl L carnitine is another form of carnitine that is particularly useful for helping to balance the parasympathetic aspect of the nervous system as it has been reported to increase muscarinic receptors. Ginkgo is also described to increase muscarinic receptor density. Ribose has been documented to raise ATP levels. Elevated levels of ATP will in turn help to generate energy to aid in the removal of glutamate from the brain.

B vitamins are crucial for nerve health. They also help to form the sulfur containing amino acids. A really good B complex is important.

42

In addition, B12 can be taken sublingually so that it is not degraded in the stomach. B12 helps with energy as well as repairs nerves. B12 is also important in helping to compensate for the MTHFr mutation that seems to be present in most of these children. It is important to take B vitamins as a complex, as it has been shown that taking a single B vitamin will deplete the levels of the other B vitamins and this occurs in a dose dependent fashion. For example, a central inflammatory mediator in other neurological inflammation is homocysteine. Lack of particular B's will increase the homocysteine levels in the blood. In the case of B vitamins a little bit of each of the specific B's with higher levels of particular B's has given the best results.

High levels of B6 or P5P can sometimes cause a child to become more "stimmy". In addition to its role in helping to convert glutamate to GABA, B6 is involved in a number of other enzymatic reactions in the body. For example, B6 helps in the metabolism of tryptophan, in its breakdown to nicotinamide. Several intermediates in this pathway, Kynurenic acid and Quinolinic acid, are involved in regulating glutamate and excitotoxins. Kynurenic acid helps to protect against excitotoxins. Quinolinic acid stimulates the glutamate receptors and can lead to excitotoxin damage. Vitamin B6 helps to convert Kynurenine to Quinolinic acid, and may therefore lead to increased levels of the excitotoxin Quinolinic acid. In children with high levels of glutamate it might therefore be wise to use small amounts of B6 and P5P. Similarly by virtue of its structure, folate contains glutamate. Again, it may be prudent to use small amounts of several derivatives of folate rather than large amounts of a single source of folate.

Another basic supplementation issue to consider is increasing the intake of Omega 3 oils (essential fatty acids like EPA and DHA) while restricting the intake of Omega 6 oils. The proper ratio of essential fats is essential for the development of healthy neurons. An imbalance exists today in virtually every one of us; Americans have a marked excess of Omega 6 oils such as soy and corn oil with a major deficiency of healthy Omega 3 oils from flax and fish. This imbalance of fatty acids increases inflammation and thus contributes to ill health. The proper levels of Omega 3 fatty acids are able to reduce the levels of inflammatory mediators including cox2, IL1 and TNF alpha. Insufficient levels of Omega 3 have been linked to everything from cancer and heart disease to our current epidemic of neurological diseases. The role of omega 3 fatty acids, in autism in particular, has been described by Dr. Andrew Stoll and others.

A healthy ratio is now believed to be 2:1 of omega 6 oils over Omega 3 in our diet. (There are some who prefer a 5:2 ratio). Researchers find that today most of us are getting a 20 fold (or greater) excess of Omega 6 over Omega 3 oils in our diet. Dr. Garry Gordon and Dr. Herb Joiner-Bey have written a book on this subject "The Omega-3 Miracle" that describes the extensive research on this vital nutrient including dramatic successes in dealing with various mental illnesses including Manic Depression and ADD. We also would limit the intake of high glycemic foods, and limit the intake of all processed foods with their heavy load of chemicals, preservatives, pesticides etc. In order to balance our Omega 3 intake, we have to lower our excessive intake of Omega 6 oils. We also need to eliminate high fructose corn syrup, which we now find everywhere, even in crackers.

Another general area to address is water. Many parents are concerned about metals or chemicals in their water supply. This is a valid concern as it is important to look at the total body burden of toxic metals and chemicals. Special bottled waters are available, however, they are often quite costly. Drinking a few bottles of "special water" daily and fulfilling the rest of the days needs with distilled water or with water purified by reverse osmosis can reach a reasonable balance. While there is no perfect solution to the water issue, if the child is supplementing with a low dose of a safe chelating agent and bathing in a chelating agent this will help to reduce toxin buildup over time. There are a wide variety of bottled

44

waters; our personal favorites are Penta water (to increase oxygenation) and Nariwa water (for the enhanced value of magnetism on the nerves).

One place where individuals can have difficulties with a supplement plan is the source/quality of the supplements and vitamins they are using. We have all heard people say "Oh, I've tried that before, it doesn't work", only to find that when they use a high quality version of that same supplement, it does in fact make a difference for them. Alternatively, there are cases where individuals were following these suggested protocols with great success, only to find that they were not doing as well when they switched to another brand of supplement, or one that was not stored properly. It is therefore important to consider "supplement quality" as an aspect of any nutritional plan. Supplements are not regulated. As a result supplement quality can vary greatly. Also, supplements can go off or spoil (similar to fresh produce) if they are not stored or shipped properly. Consequently, it is not simply a matter of supplement brand, it is also important to consider other factors, such as how it was stored (in a hot stockroom), how long it's been sitting on the shelf and how it was shipped.

Those of us practicing alternative health care did not set out with the intention of selling supplements. However, we have found that not all supplements are made under the same high standards that are necessary to have successful results. Over time we have found that it is important for you to use the proper tools to take charge of your health. One of these tools includes the use of supplements. Use good judgment in choosing your source of supplements. Please do not be guided simply by the price. The difference of a few dollars may mean the difference between a successful supplement program and one that is mediocre. (Information on specific supplements that have been "hand picked" by Dr. Amy is available from www.longevityplus.com, www.longevityplus-rna.com, www.holisticheal.com, www.holistichealth.com, and www.antiaging-systems.com).

# Step One: *Program for Neurological Inflammation*

The first step in the Program for Neurological Inflammation is removing excitotoxin triggers from the diet. This simply involves reading labels and closely monitoring food and supplement intake to avoid excitotoxins. In addition, it is important to limit the intake of calcium to prevent damage to neurons. Excess excitotoxins cause an imbalance in the flow of calcium, which leads to activation of a complex inflammatory cascade, release of inflammatory mediators and ultimately the death of neurons. Dr. Mark Neveu, President of NFAM (National Foundation of Alternative Medicine) has a wonderful and vitally important way of describing the relationship between glutamate and calcium in creating excitotoxin damage. He views glutamate as the gun, and calcium as the bullet. If both glutamate (and other excitotoxins) and calcium are kept under control, it is possible to limit the excitotoxin damage.

Most autistic children already follow a restricted diet - limiting the intake of gluten and casein. In addition, we recommend avoiding any sources of glutamate (and other excitotoxins) as well as keeping calcium under control. By adding these other dietary parameters, it is possible to limit further excitotoxin damage to the body. Calcium is kept to a minimum in the early stages of our program by limiting its ingestion and with the supplementation of magnesium and zinc. The back of this book lists various names of excitotoxins so that they can be avoided in the diet. It is also important to understand that high protein means more excitotoxins.

We recognize that the complete list of foods with excitotoxins may initially seem overwhelming. It is fortunately not necessary to eliminate every molecule, but it is necessary to limit what wc find has been the excessive intake that contributes to the overall load of glutamate and related excitotoxins. It is important to stop the inflammatory process created by these excitotoxin triggers. Halting this inflammatory cascade is achieved with a number of supplements as well as RNA-based formulas that are designed to mitigate the inflammatory process. We have found that these RNA formulas make a tremendous difference in helping to turn the tide of inflammation that even the best supplement protocols will not handle on their own.

Since one area of concern in autism is on lowering inflammation, it may be interesting to review a book by Richard Fleming MD, "Stop Inflammation Now". Although it is focused on heart disease, it, nonetheless, provides useful up to date thinking about the benefits from dramatic dietary changes along the lines of what you will be following for your child. There are still minor disagreements that your authors have with this book as well as others along the same vein, but it is useful for background reading to learn that it is increasingly clear that the American diet has set the stage for a variety of inflammatory disorders.

It is important to understand that the body is both efficient and conservative with mediators when it comes to inflammation. The very same inflammatory mediators that cause inflammation surrounding the nerves or in the gut in autism are also the culprits for the inflammation we see in heart disease, arthritis and even certain cancers.

Finally, during this first phase, it is necessary to support impaired systems and to lay the groundwork to repair and generate new neurons. This is accomplished with a variety of herbs, vitamins, and nutritional supplements that serve as antioxidants and help to reinforce the child's diet. The idea is to compensate for any imbalances in the body due to the malfunctioning of a number of organ and metabolic systems, many of which have been previously described by Dr. Jon Pangborn. The number of supplements utilized varies from approximately 5 to 50 or more, depending on the severity and the number of the imbalances in an individual child. The systems or imbalances that may require supplementation include the pancreas, the intestinal tract, excessive acid production in the stomach, the liver, hormonal imbalances, thyroid, adrenals, and neurotransmitter imbalances among others. This may seem like a lot of supplements, and in some cases it is. However, the ultimate goal is the reversal of accumulated damage. Nerve damage is a process; by the time an individual recognizes that they have neurological problems, more than 50% of their neurons may have been damaged causing obvious neurological symptoms. It takes time and commitment in order to halt and reverse this process. How long does it take to grow a new neuron? No one really knows. For years it was widely believed that it did not happen at all, but we now know that it does happen. What we do know is that when we have an individual who commits to their program and stays with it, together we are able to achieve incredible results. Remember, this is a marathon, not a sprint.

The suggested supplementation protocol is broken into categories. It is not necessary to take every supplement in every category. However, depending upon the severity of an individual case of autism, you may find it necessary to use every supplement listed. It is always possible that a particular child may be sensitive to an individual herb or supplement. It is best for this reason to add supplements slowly to the program, allowing several days to be certain that the newly added supplements agree with the child before progressing to add additional new supplements. Yes, it will take a while to introduce all the new supplements. It is important to remember to be calm and patient, and not feel rushed to get through the program.

An alternative to slowly adding supplements and allowing several days to determine a child's reaction to a particular supplement is to take advantage of energy testing. There are a number of qualified individuals who will provide energy testing for you and your child to determine which are the most appropriate supplements for your child's individual program. There are also a number of reputable sources for EAV equipment for home or office use that will aid in supplement choices based on an individual child's particular needs. Many EAV practitioners also practice homeopathy. The use of homeopathy for autism works well in conjunction with the protocol we have described. Our protocol has not been found to interfere with the use of homeopathic drugs, and the use of homeopathics may have a synergistic effect with this program.

The suggested dosage on any supplement listed in our protocol is 1/2 to 1 whole unless otherwise noted. This will be <u>well below</u> the dosage suggested on the labels of the bottles. The approach is to try to rebalance a number of pathways in the body simultaneously. If you begin to think about the body as a roadway system, imagine that you are supplementing the main road, the side roads, and the back roads all at the same time. This requires a <u>small</u> amount of a <u>large</u> number of supplements. This is the way the body is accustomed to working, having multiple pathways and feedback systems to get to the same point.

## Step One: *Suggested Protocol for Neurological Inflammation*

Vitamins/ minerals/ antioxidants to lay the nutritional groundwork:
Complete Vitamin & Ultra Antioxidant
Vitamin D
Vitamin C (Beyond C)
Cell Food
Primal Defense
Vitamin E +mixed tocopherols
Potassium chloride (depending on levels)
Liquid Selenium drops
Liquid Molybdenum drops
Iodine (depending on levels)
DHEA (depending on testosterone levels) supports new nerves
Nerve Calm RNA NutriSwitch Formula (2X/day or as needed)
Health Foundation RNA NutriSwitch Formula (2X/day or as needed)

Stress RNA NutriSwitch Formula (2X/day or as needed)
HyperImmune RNA NutriSwitch Formula (2X/day or as needed)
Behavior RNA NutriSwitch Formula (2X/day or as needed)
Bowel RNA NutriSwitch Formula (2X/day or as needed)
Stomach pH RNA NutriSwitch Formula (2X/day or as needed)

Support liver health/ increase glutathione/ increase sulfur:
Milk thistle
B complex + SAMe
Alpha lipoic acid
Taurine
Broccoli
Rosemary
Garlic
Sublingual Glutathione
Oral GSH Glutathione
Glutathione Shampoo
Glutathione Toothpaste
(some parents prefer IV glutathione)
Glucosamine/ MSM
Chondroitin Sulfate
N-acetyl cysteine w/ Quercetin
Vitamin C (with Rose Hips) (500mg c for every 250 mg NAC)
Dandelion root
Carnitine
Cod Liver Oil
Ora-Liv
Creams (transdermal):
    Glutathione cream
    Magnesium sulfate cream
    Alpha lipoic acid cream
    Glucosamine/ MSM cream

Supplements to aid in protection from excess calcium:
        Magnesium
        Vinpocetine
        Zinc (25-40mg/day)

Supplements to aid in the balance of glutamate and GABA:
        Branched Chain Amino Acids (ONLY leu/ileu/val)
        (discontinue immediately if urines smells like "maple syrup")
        Pycnogenol
        Grape seed extract
        GABA
        Sublingual GABA Calm/ Glycine
        Sublingual methylcobalamin (B12)
        Sublingual cyanocobalamine (B12)
        Sublingual hydroxycobalamin (B12)
        ZEN
        L-Theanine
        Taurine
        Cats Claw
        Trehalose

Supplements to Support the Pancreas:
        Ora-Pancreas
        Vitamin K
        Super Digestive Enzymes-with meals
        Ayur-Gymnema

Decrease yeast/ repopulate GI tract/ decrease E.coli and Strep:
        Super Digestive Enzymes-with meals
        Ultra Dairy enzymes-with meals
        Kyodophilus-with meals
        Oregon grape
        Myrrh Gum
        Neem
        Goldenseal
        Uva Ursi (limited use)

Cranberry - chewable
Oregamax
Caprylic acid
Stomach pH RNA NutriSwitch Formula (with meals)
Bowel RNA NutriSwitch Formula (2X/day or as needed)
Candex
Lactoferrin
Suprema Dophilus
Grapefruit Seed extract
Inuflora
ARA6

Support to Reducing Stims:
Nettle
Behavior RNA NutriSwitch Formula (2X/day or as needed)
Stress RNA NutriSwitch Formula (2X/day or as needed)
Inositol or IP6

Support Membrane Fluidity:
Phosphatidyl serine or Pedia-active chewable
Essential Fatty Acid Mixture
Neuromins (DHA)
Policosanol

Aid in helping inflammation around nerves:
Health Foundation RNA NutriSwitch (2X/day or as needed)
HyperImmune RNA NutriSwitch (2X/day or as needed)
Boswellia
Curcumin

Supplements to support energy/ protect the brain:
CoQ 10
NADH
Ginkgo Biloba
Oxydrene
Idebenone

ATP
Vinpocetine
L-Carnitine
Melatonin

Support proper sugar glycosylation/ balance Zinc/ Copper:
Carnosine
Vitamin K
Rosemary
EDTA (just 1X/day at this stage)
Molybdenum

Supplements to support the gut:
Curcumin
Slippery Elm
Colostrum
Glucosamine/MSM
Mastica Gum
Bowel RNA NutriSwitch Formula (2X/day or as needed)
Slippery Elm

Supplements to aid in Constipation:
Artichoke
Yellow Dock
Cascara Sagrada
Aloe Vera
Magnesium
Cod Liver oil
Rhubarb

*Note:* *If supplements are listed in more than one category the intention is to take the supplement only once a day. They are listed in each category to give a sense of the multiple uses of the individual supplements. These supplements can be purchased through Holistic Health Consultants, L.L.C (www.holisticheal.com) and Longevity Plus-RNA, L.L.C (www.longevityplus-rna.com).*

## Step Two: *Program for Toxin Elimination*

The next phase of the protocol helps to remove toxins from the body. This is the "elimination" part of the program. Brooks and his colleagues have demonstrated a strategy to eliminate chronic stores of retrovirus in the body that serve as a source for renewed viral infection. Their work has shown that activating the latently infected cells makes them susceptible to therapy and depletes the bulk of the reservoir of infected cells. Expanding on this philosophy, we have found that it is possible to support the body with supplements that should help to eradicate the latent reservoir of virus. As the virus is eliminated, we see a release of stored metals from the body. Supplements are added during this phase to help eliminate both chronic virus and metals.

Detoxification can be very stressful on the body. It is therefore important to allow sufficient time for Step One before progressing to Step Two. Organ systems should be functioning better, the "stims" should be down, there should be better eye contact, better sleep, and an improvement in the bowels and absorption before progressing to Step Two. The comprehensive supplementation program that was used in Step One should be continued to ensure that the immune system and other organs are well supported during the elimination process. Any new supplements in the Detoxification part of the program should be added in the same way those new supplements were added in Step One. Again, it is not necessary to take every supplement in every category. However, depending upon the severity of the individual you may find it necessary to use every supplement listed. It is always possible that a particular child may be sensitive to an individual herb or supplement. It is best for this reason to add supplements slowly to the program, allowing several days to be certain that the newly added supplements agree with the child before progressing to add additional new supplements. Yes, it will take a while to introduce all the new supplements. Again, this is a marathon, not a sprint! The suggested dosage on any supplement is 1/2 to 1 whole capsule or tablet unless otherwise noted. This will be well below the dosage suggested on the labels of the bottles.

**WAIT** to begin 5 methyl folate (Folapro), intrinsic B12, nucleotides, folinic (or Actfol), and Metals NutriSwitch RNA Formulas until the rest of the supplements to support detoxification have been added and are well tolerated. **THEN** begin to add 1/4 to 1/2 of 5 methyl folate, intrinsic B12, the nucleotides, and 1/8 capsule of folinic. The role of the Folapro, intrinsic B12, nucleotides and folinic is to compensate for the MTHFr mutation. This will open up the pathway, and in doing so will allow the proper expansion of T cells to aid in viral elimination. It is for this precise reason that we ask you to WAIT to add these supplements, until the body has had a chance to rebalance in Step One, and then have the immune support necessary in Step Two before beginning a detoxification process.

There seems to be a tremendous amount of confusion in the literature concerning 5 methyl folate. Only 5 methyl folate will bypass the MTHFr mutation; 5 formyl folate has other advantages, but it will not bypass the mutation. In order to go from 5 formyl THF to 5 methyl THF requires MTHFr. The product called Folapro is clearly 5 methyl THF. There are products on the market labeled as folinic acid that are 5 formyl THF and others labeled folinic that are 5 methyl THF. Given the confusion, it is safer to use a product based on the chemical formula, rather than to use it based on its name on the label.

Once the 5 methyl folate (Folapro), intrinsic B12, nucleotides, folinic (or Actfol) have been added and well tolerated, it is time to begin with Metal I NutriSwitch RNA Formula. Start with 1/2 dropper only 1X /day. You will continue at this low dosage for 2-3 weeks. "Overmethylated children" represent the exception to the above-suggested dosages. Methylation is necessary to prevent the expression of viral genes that have been inserted into the body's DNA. Children who are overmethylated may therefore have lower viral loads than children who are undermethylators. It is better to err on the side of "less is better" with respect to methylation with these children. Use 1/8 to 1/4 of the 5 methyl folate, intrinsic B12 and nucleotides for overmethylators, and use between 1/4 to 1/2 dropper of the RNA NutriSwitch Metal formulas for these children.

Watch for signs of detoxification. These may include a rash, mild fever, mood changes, crankiness, and loose bowels. Occasionally children will vomit during this phase for no apparent reason, and then quickly resume their previous activity or even sit down for something to eat. This is all a part of the detoxification process. Several of the other NutriSwitch formulas may help to alleviate some of the discomfort associated with detoxification. It is fine to increase the dosage of the Health Foundation NutriSwitch RNA Formula, the Stress NutriSwitch RNA Formula, the Behavior NutriSwitch RNA Formula, and the Nerve Calm NutriSwitch RNA Formula. You may also want to try one or more of the Mood NutriSwitch RNA formulas if your child is particularly moody during detoxification. If you experience more severe symptoms of detoxification, discontinue Step Two immediately. If you have questions during this phase of the program (or any other phases) please take advantage of the www.autismanswer.com website for online discussions and questions. In addition, it is recommended that you work with a qualified practitioner while following this protocol.

As you begin to experience detoxification, you will notice the urine getting darker. This can be monitored by weekly urine toxic metal tests. It is fine to take random spot urines some time in the mid afternoon. It is best to pick a day and time of the week to monitor and stick with that day and time weekly (i.e. Tuesday at 2:00 pm). You will notice that the creatinine numbers on the urine test will increase, as the urine gets darker. It is postulated that this represents viral detoxification in the urine. Eventually the urine will get lighter, almost clear. This is often when the metals begin to be excreted. You will be able to visualize this by continuing to take weekly urine samples. Over this time period you can begin to gradually increase the frequency of the Metal I NutriSwitch RNA Formula. After 2-3 weeks of 1/2 dropper once a day, you can gradually increase to 1/2 dropper 2X/day for several days, then to 3X/day, up to 7-8X/day. As you increase the dosage of the Metal I NutriSwitch RNA Formula you will notice increases in the creatinine (or color of the urine) followed by increases in the metal excretion. After you have reached a dosage of Metal I NutriSwitch RNA Formula of 7-8 X/day for several weeks, and you are no longer seeing any excretion of metals, drop back to a maintenance dose of 1/2 dropper 1X/day. Occasionally, a child will appear to be almost "stuck" at this phase of detoxification. The urine remains dark, the creatinine continues to be high, and a very low but steady excretion of metals are seen on the urine tests.  This is okay; every child is unique and may respond somewhat differently to the program.  Just hang in there, don't feel rushed, and continue with the program until you finally see the urine clear and the metals begin to flow.  While the average time for using Metal I at 7-8X/day is only a few weeks, we have seen children who required several months at this point. Realize that this program is not an "all or none" phenomena. You will see gradual changes as you progress through the program.

Once you have finished with Metals I, it is a good idea to give the body a rest for 2-4 weeks before going on to Metal II NutriSwitch RNA Formula. It may be tempting to rush through the program once you begin to see metals and virus flowing. However, it is much easier on the system to give it time to rest between detoxification. In addition, it is often normal to see regressions in behavior and speech during detoxification. This can be scary for the parents. Giving a break between phases allows the behavior and the language to "bounce back", which is reassuring for everyone involved. With all of these caveats in mind, when you are ready, you can progress to Metal II NutriSwitch RNA Formula.

This next phase of detoxification proceeds in basically the same fashion as the first phase. Continue with a maintenance dose of

Metal I NutriSwitch RNA Formula at 1/2 dropper 1X/day. You can then add the Metal II NutriSwitch RNA Formula, starting with 1/2 dropper only 1X /day. You will continue at this low dosage for 2-3 weeks. After 2-3 weeks of 1/2 dropper once a day, you can gradually increase to 1/2 dropper 2X/day for several days, then to 3X/day, up to 7-8X/day. As you increase the dosage of the Metal II NutriSwitch RNA Formula you will again notice increases in the creatinine (or color of the urine) followed by increases in the metal excretion. After you have reached a dosage of Metal II NutriSwitch RNA Formula of 7-8X/day and you are no longer seeing any excretion of metals, drop back to a maintenance dose of 1/2 dropper 1X/day. At this point you will be using a maintenance dose of both Metal I NutriSwitch RNA Formula and Metal II NutriSwitch RNA Formula. Urines can be monitored during this second phase of detoxification as they were during the first phase. Again, at this point it is a good idea to give the body a rest for 2-4 weeks before going on to Metal III NutriSwitch RNA Formula.

The third phase of detoxification proceeds basically the same as the first two phases. Continue with a maintenance dose of Metal I NutriSwitch RNA Formula, and Metal II NutriSwitch RNA Formula at 1/2 dropper 1X/day for each. You can then add the Metal III NutriSwitch RNA Formula, starting with 1/2 dropper only 1X /day. You will continue at this low dosage for 2-3 weeks. After 2-3 weeks of 1/2 dropper once a day, you can gradually increase to 1/2 dropper 2X/day for several days, then to 3X/day, up to 7-8X/day. As you increase the dosage of the Metal III NutriSwitch RNA Formula you will again notice increases in the creatinine (or color of the urine) followed by increases in the metal excretion. After you have reached a dosage of Metal III NutriSwitch RNA Formula of 7-8X/day for several weeks and you are no longer seeing any excretion of metals, drop back to a maintenance dose of 1/2 dropper 1X/day. At this point you will be using a maintenance dose of both Metal I NutriSwitch RNA Formula and Metal II NutriSwitch RNA Formula and Metal III NutriSwitch RNA Formula. Urines can be monitored during this third phase of detoxification as they were during the first two phases. Again, at this point it is a good idea to give the body a rest for 2-4 weeks before going on to Metal IV NutriSwitch RNA Formula.

Weekly urine tests can get expensive, although the feedback is always gratifying for the parents. One trick is to watch for the color of the urine to get dark, and then get clear again. Simply send in the clear samples to try to get a measure of the metal excretion. This will not monitor creatinine and potential viral excretion, and you may miss some metals, but it will be easier on the budget.

After a sufficient rest following Metals I, II, III it is time to progress to Metals IV. At this point you will be using a maintenance dose of Metal I NutriSwitch RNA Formula and Metal II NutriSwitch RNA Formula and Metal III NutriSwitch RNA Formula. Initially the Metal IV formulation can be used topically for the best results. At this point we are trying to enhance any metal detoxification through the skin. Urine tests can be continued but will most likely show little or no new metal excretion. Stool toxic analysis has proven useful at this stage of detoxification. In addition the skin rash can be more visible at this time. Frequent baths are a good idea at this stage of detoxification. The bath should contain EDTA (Beyond Clean) and may also contain malic acid, and oatmeal or Aveeno to relieve itching. The Health Foundation NutriSwitch RNA as well as the HyperImmune NutriSwitch Formulas may also be useful used topically at this point. In addition, the Topical Skin Formula is also helpful, as well as any topical creams including glutathione, horse chestnut, aloe, MSM. Saunas may be helpful to accelerate detoxification through the skin. The use of saunas to accelerate toxin release has been thoroughly described by Dr. Stephen Edelson. Metals IV can be applied topically as a cosmetic prior to taking a sauna to enhance absorption.

After 2-3 weeks of topical use of Metals IV it is time to progress to more systemic use. This next phase of detoxification using Metals IV proceeds in basically the same fashion as the previous phases.

Continue with the maintenance doses of Metals I, II, III NutriSwitch RNA Formulas at 1/2 dropper 1X/day. You can then add the Metal IV NutriSwitch RNA Formula, starting with 1/2 dropper only 1X /day. You will continue at this low dosage for 2-3 weeks. After 2-3 weeks of 1/2 dropper once a day, you can gradually increase to 1/2 dropper 2X/day for several days, then to 3X/day, up to 7-8X/day. After you have reached a dosage of Metal IV NutriSwitch RNA Formula of 7-8X/day and you are no longer seeing any excretion of metals, drop back to a maintenance dose of 1/2 dropper 1X/day. During this final phase of detoxification metals are often excreted in the stool as well as the urine. Stools should be monitored during this final phase of detoxification.

There have been mixed reports concerning the use of Vitamin A to aid in eradicating chronic viral infection. Some parents choose to add 100,000 IU of Vitamin A every other day for a period of 2 weeks as a concentrated approach to aiding in recovery from virus. In addition, some protocols use prescription antivirals, such as Valtrex in conjunction with the Metal IV portion of the detoxification program. It is worth considering the use of Valtrex, and Metals I, II, III prior to, or in conjunction with the use of Depakane (valproic acid). Valproic acid can be used to treat seizures. There is literature to suggest that valproic acid may exacerbate measles viral infection. Subsequent research has found the combination of Valtrex in conjunction with depakane to be beneficial.

It is normal to see rashes, a mild fever, and regression in behavior during detoxification. Occasionally, parents have reported that their child may vomit, for no particular reason, during this phase, and then calmly resume their activity or even sit down for something to eat with no ill effects. This may be part of the detoxification process. At any point during the detoxification program that you are concerned about behaviors, the extent of detoxification, rashes, fever, or other physical symptoms simply stop the program and those symptoms will subside in several days. You can go back to the program at any point and restart. Simply remember to begin again at a dose of 1X/day, and gradually work your way up.

Some parents like to accelerate the detoxification program. This can be accomplished by increasing the dosage of some of the other supplements. For instance, during Step One (Program for Neurological Inflammation) we used a maintenance dose of EDTA once a day, and additional garlic once a day. During Step Two, the detoxification part of the program the dosages of EDTA and garlic can be gradually increased to aid in accelerating the process. Also don't forget to continue with nightly baths using the EDTA Beyond Clean formula. This will aid in detoxification through the skin. A number of parents have also chosen to combine saunas with the detoxification portion of the protocol, again to help accelerate the detoxification.

It is important to keep the concept of the total body burden of metals and chemicals in mind during detoxification. There has understandably been a tremendous emphasis on mercury with respect to elimination. However, toxic levels of lead, aluminum and other metals can be just as dangerous. Cadmium has the ability to enhance the toxic level of lead, making lower levels of lead more toxic in the presence of cadmium. We have seen children excrete exceedingly high levels of uranium and tin (see sample detox data). One can only speculate as to the cumulative effects of these metal levels in conjunction with only minor levels of mercury.

We therefore need to consider the synergistic total burden on the body. We have noted some interesting kinetics in terms of metal excretion in urine. We have observed that nickel is often excreted prior to mercury, and that cadmium excretion often precedes that of lead. The kinetics of metal excretion will continue to be clarified in the future, and we will adjust this protocol to reflect future findings. We continue to evolve our detoxification protocol, and an additional detoxification step, Metals V, is currently under development.

# Step Two: *Suggested Protocol to Support Detoxification*

Vitamins/ minerals/ antioxidants to lay the nutritional groundwork:
    Cell Food
    Primal Defense
    Selenium
    Molybdenum
    Complete Vitamin & Ultra Antioxidant
    Vitamin D
    Nerve Calm RNA NutriSwitch Formula
    Health Foundation RNA NutriSwitch Formula
    Stress RNA NutriSwitch Formula
    HyperImmune RNA NutriSwitch Formula
    Behavior RNA NutriSwitch Formula
    Bowel RNA NutriSwitch Formula
    Stomach pH RNA NutriSwitch Formula

Supplements to Support Viral Detoxification:
    Metal I RNA NutriSwitch Formula (progress to Metals II, III, and IV)
    FolaPro (5 methyl folate)
    Intrinsic B12/Folate
    Folinic
    Nucleotides
    Elderberry
    Garlic (start with 1X/day, may increase up to 6X/day)
    Policosanol
    Glutathione  (1X/day, then increase to 4 or more per day)
    L-Lysine
    Melissa
    Moducare (start 1X in AM and 1X in PM, increase to 4X/day)
    EDTA (start with 1X/day, may increase to 4-6X/day)
    Beyond Clean EDTA bath- nightly
    Colostrum (start with 1X/day, then increase to 2-3X/day)
    Alpha Lipoic Acid
    Vitamin C (Beyond C)

Synthetic B1
Transfer Factor
Cats Claw
Aloe Vera
Quercetin
Proline
Licorice

Supplements to Support the Immune System/ Increase White Cells:
Transfer Factor
IP6
MGN3
Mycoceutics (mushrooms/beta glucan)
Pau d Arco
Ayur-Guggulipid
Myrrh Gum
Fenugreek
SerenAid *(start with 1/4 per day, increase to 1/2 or 1X/day)*
Lactoferrin (every other day)
L-Theanine

Supplements to Help Support the Liver/ Pancreas/ Thymus/ Spleen:
Ora -Triplex
Immuno-Forte
Ora-Liv
Ora-Pancreas
Cod Liver Oil
SAMe
B Complex
Ora-Kidney

Support Oxygenation/ Alkalinity to Limit Viral Growth:
Oxydrene
Penta water
ATP

Cell Food
Ionic Breeze (Sharper Image)
pH Kit and balancing for alkaline pH

Optional:
Vitamin A (100,000 IU every other day for 2 weeks)
Valtrex

**Note:** *If supplements are listed in more than one category the intention is to take the supplement only once a day.  They are listed in each category to give a sense of the multiple uses of the individual supplements.  These supplements can be purchased through Holistic Health Consultants, L.L.C (www.holisticheal.com), Longevity Plus, L.L.C (www.longevityplus.com), and Longevity Plus-RNA, L.L.C (www.longevityplus-rna.com).*

# Step Three: *Program for Nerve Growth & Myelination*

This is the phase that everyone has been waiting for. Unfortunately, there is still a bit more waiting even during this phase. It can take up to nine months to remyelinate the nerves that have been demyelinated from virus, metals, and other assaults to the system. Once the nerves are remyelinated they are finally in a position to begin the "pruning" process. This also takes time. The exception to this is children who are "over methylators". This process will occur much more rapidly for children who tend to be over methylated.

The methylation pathway is also tied into the pathways for neurotransmitters. As a result, you may see changes in mood and behaviors as you go through this phase. Initially many parents will comment that the child is "no longer autistic" but "acts more like a child with ADD". This makes sense as dopamine has been implicated in ADD as well as in the methylation process. The Mood RNA NutriSwitch Formulas can be very helpful at this stage. There are three Mood Formulas. Depending on the particular child one or more of these Formulas may be helpful. A good starting point is to use 1/2 dropper of one of the formulas for several days and make a decision on that formula before switching to a different formula or adding a second formula for a combined effect. Also, some parents have seen great things with small amounts of supplements containing natural dopamine.

At this point, depending on the calcium levels seen on a urine essential element test, you may want to look at adding calcium back. It will aid in neurotransmission; however, too much calcium can still be a problem. One approach is to use a calcium/magnesium/vitamin D/vitamin K supplement, and substitute it for the individual magnesium, vitamin D and vitamin K supplements. Again, this will vary depending on the child and on the level of calcium in the system.

It is possible to accelerate the myelination process somewhat by using higher dosages of some of the supplements that support myelination. Some parents have used up to four SAMe per day with two B complex. In addition, they have used two curcumin and doubled up on some of the other methylating agents. While this may speed up the process, watch carefully for potential side effects such as mood swings or vision issues. If this occurs, back off on the dosages. Do NOT increase the levels of 5 methyl folate, intrinsic, folinic, or the nucleotides. Due to the MTHFr mutation in virtually all of the children, this could create problems. You are better off to just keep the door open on this MTHFr pathway, rather than flooding it with supplementation. B12 deserves special mention in terms of dosage. So far, according to published work by Dr. Neubrander, no toxic doses of B12 have been found. The more the better seems to be what parents are finding. In some cases going to highly elevated doses of B12 (50 milligrams and above) has helped to stimulate speech in children that were apraxic. However, it is always possible that your child will be the one child who will react adversely to high doses of B12. Again, progress slowly, use caution, and consult with your health care practitioner when utilizing this or any other program. Children who are "overmethylators" are the exception. These children cannot tolerate high doses of any methylating agents, so caution and low doses should be used when supplementing these children with methylating agents.

The major focus of this final phase of the program involves supplements to support remyelination of the nerves and supplements to foster left/right communication in the brain. Many of the supplements used in the previous phases can be discontinued at this time. The approach to discontinuing supplements should be very similar to the approach used to add supplements. Eliminate several supplements at a time, and then wait to be sure that you are not seeing regressions as a result of discontinuing supplements. Go back to the categories listed in Step One, and try to keep in some support from each category. Even though we may have detoxified virus and metals, there are still many of the underlying factors discussed in the earlier portions of this book. The idea is to keep enough supplementation in the program to prevent this entire process from happening all over again. No one wants that to happen! So, while you may be tempted to only use the supplements listed in Step Three for Nerve Growth and Myelination, remember where you have been. It is a lot easier to give a little bit of a large number of supplements daily, then to run the risk of glutamate, viral and metal toxin buildup occurring again.

You may want to consider incorporating the use of magnetic therapy at this time. The basic premise for the use of magnetic devices is that the human body responds to the influence of the Earth's magnetic field. However, the strength of this field has decreased over time. In certain individuals this lack of magnetism can cause deficiencies, which can be improved by the use of external applications of magnetic fields.

Applications of magnetic fields have been successful in diverse situations, affecting specific chemical reactions (Grenoble High Magnetic Field Laboratory and the Max Planck Society) to the reduction of pain. In laboratory animals, magnets can act like a switch to open or constrict blood vessels, potentially increasing blood flow to damaged tissues. Pulsed electromagnetic fields have been shown to reduce bone resorption, and increase vascularization and bone formation. The use of magnetized water (Nariwa) is reported to aid in the excretion of mercury.

While Dr. Yasko has not found the use of magnetic energy to enhance metal excretion, she has seen a significant discernable affect on more subtle cognitive function. This would agree with recent work by Dr. Dean Bonlie, which has found electromagnetic therapy to be safe and effective for a wide range of neurological problems and that it may help to regenerate and repair damaged nerves and enhance the body's natural stem cells. Magnetic energy may also increase the oxygen carrying capacity of the blood, improving the assimilation of nutrients and oxygenation of tissues. The use of Nariwa magnetized water, and Penta oxygenated water may also be useful adjuncts to any program to enhance nerve growth and demyelination.

This is also a point where it would make sense to begin to integrate therapies that enhance nerve growth and maturation. The March 2004 issue of the Journal of Neuroscience describes significant increases in the levels of BDNF (brain derived neurotrophic factor) depending on the environment; an enriched environment fostered higher levels of this factor. BDNF promotes neuronal growth and survival and regulates communication between neurons. Dr. Cheri Florence, a medical speech/language pathologist, has described tremendous personal success with her own son. She has made use of strategies, which may help to create an enriched environment, by taking advantage of enhanced visual thinking to help promote language.

Dr. David Steenblock, Dr. Barbara Brewitt and Dr. Luis Aguilar have pioneered the direct use of some of these brain growth factors for stroke as well as autism, among others. Insulin like growth factor (IGF) has been found to stimulate enzymes in the methylation pathway in addition to its effects on neural development. Fibroblast growth factor (FgF) has also been found to have activities beyond its effects on nerve growth; FgF has been reported to increase dopamine levels, as well as to decrease seizure activity.

Dr. Edward Traub has developed CI (constraint induced) Movement therapy, which has proven to expedite recovery times after stroke. The basis of the therapy is helping the brain to overcome "learned non-use". Some of these therapies may be applicable to autism in the future to help to accelerate recovery after the biochemical imbalances have been addressed.

Music therapy has been reported to be successful in helping to enhance speech in children. A number of scientific journals have found that music affects regions of the brain involved in cognitive, affective and mnemonic processing. The entire July 2003 issue of

Nature Neuroscience was devoted to music and neuroscience, as was the March 2004 issue of the New York Academy of Sciences magazine. Recent research from the University of London suggests that many autistic children have outstanding abilities in tone memory and discrimination. Music therapy may be an avenue worth exploring to help to enhance language skills during this point of the program.

## Step Three: *Suggested Protocol to Support Nerve Growth & Myelination*

General Vitamin/ Organ Support:
> Complete Vitamin & Ultra Antioxidant
> Liquid Trace Minerals
> Ora-Liv
> Ora-Pancreas
> Ora-Triplex
> Immuno-Forte
> Cod Liver Oil
> Zinc
> Potassium chloride (depending on levels)
> Nerve Calm RNA NutriSwitch Formula
> Health Foundation RNA NutriSwitch Formula
> Stress RNA NutriSwitch Formula
> Nerve Coat RNA NutriSwitch Formula
> Behavior RNA NutriSwitch Formula
> Bowel RNA NutriSwitch Formula
> Stomach pH RNA NutriSwitch Formula

Support Nutrient Transport to Brain (taken with supplements):
> Vitamin C (Beyond C)

Support Methylation (increases myelin):
> Curcumin
> SAMe
> B12 (balance of methyl/cyano/hydroxy cobalamine)

Intrinsic B12/Folate
FolaPro (5 Methyl Folate)
Folinic
Nucleotides
DMG
B Complex
Selenium (up to 100-200mcg/day incl. Complete Vitamins)
Amino Care amino acids
MSM

Support Myelination/Cell Membranes Fluidity:
DHA (100-600mg/day)
Phosphatidyl serine
Nerve Coat RNA NutriSwitch (1/2 dropper 2X/day or as needed)
EFA
Policosanol
Chondroitin sulfate (high MW)
Glucosamine sulfate

Help limit ROS, which trigger macrophage digestion of myelin:
CoQ10
Alpha Lipoic Acid
Idebenone
Vitamin E +mixed tocopherols

Limit macrophage digestion of myelin (MAY be an issue for phenol sensitive):
Flavinoids:
Lutein/Bilberry
Quercetin
Pycnogenol
Grape Seed extract
Elderberry
Cranberry
Green Tea or L-Theanine

Support New Nerve growth/ support nerves:
Ashwaganda
SAMe
B12
Milk thistle
B complex
Colostrum
IGF
FGF
HGH
Taurine
Ora-Placenta
Ginkgo Biloba
Carnosine
Rosemary
DHEA (monitor with hormone test)
Synthetic B1 (benfotiamine)
Shark liver oil (nervonic acid)
Vitamin K (or vit d/k/ca/mg depending on calcium levels)
Vitamin D  (or vit d/k/ca/mg depending on calcium levels)
Magnesium  (or vit d/k/ca/mg depending on calcium levels)
Calcium- *DEPENDING ON CALCIUM LEVELS*
L-Tyrosine
Glutathione
Choline, or lecithin, or huperzine (depending on the child)

Supplements to support progesterone for nerve growth:
GABA
Sublingual GABA Calm/ Glycine
Zen

Support Oxygenation/ Energy for New Nerve Growth:
Oxydrene
ATP
Carnitine/acetyl-carnitine
Vinpocetine

NADH
Cell Food
Magnetico Magnetic Mattress (north only, 20 gauss)
Body Fields OMT Magnopro
Ionic Breeze (Sharper Image)
Penta water
Hyperbaric oxygen
Nariwa water

Supplements to Support Moods:
Mood-S NutriSwitch Formula
Mood-D NutriSwitch Formula
Mood & Focus NutriSwitch Formula
Dopa 400

Support language:
DMG
Fenugreek (start with 1X/day increase to 3X/day)
Gotu Kola
Bacopa
Piracetam
B12-cyano/methyl/hydroxy cobalamin
Black Cohosh
Dong Quai
Indole 3 Carbinol (discontinue if a fish odor from the body)
Methylation Support RNA NutriSwitch Formula
Spinal Nerve Support RNA NutriSwitch Formula

Supplements to support left/ right communication:
Gotu Kola
Bacopa
Nootropics:
Piracetam
Aniracetam
Fenugreek
Creatine

Supplements to keep virus in check <u>IF still an issue</u>:
    Transfer Factor
    Moducare (may increase gamma interferon)
    Glutathione
    Metals I, II, III, IV RNA NutriSwitch Formulas

***Note:** If supplements are listed in more than one category the intention is to take the supplement only once a day.  They are listed in each category to give a sense of the multiple uses of the individual supplements.  These supplements can be purchased through Holistic Health Consultants, L.L.C (www.holisticheal.com), Longevity Plus, L.L.C (www.longevityplus.com), and Longevity Plus-RNA, L.L.C (www.longevityplus-rna.com).*

# Conclusion: *A Ship in the Storm*

*"At 13 months we were traveling with our son in Europe and people would stop us and say, "Look how he looks at you, the love in his eyes." By 18 months he no longer knew who we were, was unable to look at us and had lost all his language (he was speaking English and Spanish words). The pediatrician told us "Yes, 18 months is when Autism/PDD begins".*

*As parents, pregnant with twin boys at the time, we began frantically researching and traveling all over the US, meeting with DAN doctors, going to conferences etc. The physicians we met with, all had a piece of the puzzle and our son began to show improvements but we were far from recovery.*

*At 3 years old we still had no language so we taught Matthew to sign for things he needed. He still had many sensory issues; repetitive behavior couldn't sleep at night and would have terrible tantrums.*

*At the DAN conference in Boston 2002 I met some mothers from New York and they invited me to a meeting they have once a month at Jacobi Hospital. My husband and I went and we sat next to a mom who was talking about the success she was having with this "Dr. Amy" in Maine. She had been through the circuit of DAN doctors that we were now going to, and told us "Amy has figured it out".*

*I called Amy the next day and got an appointment within the next few weeks. We feel blessed because now we would have to wait quite some time, and that is why this book is so important.*

*Amy spent two hours on the phone with us on our initial consult. My husband is an MD and he was blown away by Amy's intelligence and dedication. He was also a bit skeptical about the supplements she was recommending because he was not trained that way. We began her protocol anyway.*

*Matthew continued to recover everyday with Amy's protocol; we also used Dr. Gordon's EDTA to slowly chelate him. In July of 2003, Amy sent us the detoxification phase of the protocol. One month later Matthew began excreting high levels of mercury and other metals. By the middle of September, Matthew walked in our kitchen and asked in a perfect sentence "could he have a glass of water". We almost fell on the floor.*

*Matthew just turned 5 in June 2004. He just graduated from Preschool, and he was the star of the show. He has incredible language and loves to play with other kids. He no longer has repetitive behavior and will be going to kindergarten in September. He loves to have sleepovers with his friends and with his cousins.*

*We are about 95% recovered from that deep dark world that Matthew was stuck in. We are now in the fine tuning phase. Our twin boys are now 2 years 7 months. We now have three healthy beautiful little boys.*

*We are so happy that Amy and Dr. Gordon have decided to publish a book on the protocols so other families can get started. It is a long but rewarding journey for everyone involved. Amy will continue to research and educate the parents to give them the knowledge to recover the children. Through this process she has rescued Matthew and saved my other two sons from going down that dreadful dark ally. We are truly grateful to her."*

Marilyn M. and Dr. John M., Parents of Matthew, age 5

Now you have read through the protocols and can't wait to get started. That is excellent. Any parent or physician reading this should be excited and hopeful. This protocol has been a tremendous benefit to a number of children. It has worked for children of all ages, and no, this protocol does not require that your child be less than 5 years old. Individuals up to 30 years of age have seen benefits from this program. However, it is not a magic bullet. For most children there is no magic bullet. It is a matter of perseverance, and slowly working your way through the program to gradually reverse the layers of damage, and put all of the complex pieces back together and in working order. Yes, it can be done, and it has been done. There are always the "quick fix" kids; the ones that need only a few supplements or just the first phase of the detoxification program to be on their way to recovery. We all hear about those cases, and it seems like everyone except YOUR child falls into that category. Well, the reality is that most children do not fall into the quick fix category. But there is hope for every child. So, take a deep breath, get ready for the marathon, pace yourself, but above all else don't give up on your children.

One way to think about neurological inflammation is like a ship that is drifting out to sea, being carried further and further from shore by the tide. Out of nowhere, a rope is thrown to that ship. First, all that happens is the ship stops moving out to sea with the tide. It seems like nothing is happening and all is still lost. However, the very fact that the ship is no longer moving, that it is staying in place, means that the movement out to sea has been stopped, that the direction is reversed, and the progression of the disease has been halted. Then slowly the ship begins to move back toward the shore. It moves very slowly because it moves against the tide working to pull it back out to sea. Over time, the ship moves closer and closer to the land until finally, when you least expect it, there it is, safe on the shore. Hold on tight to your rope, don't lose hope; it truly is possible to get your children well.

*With love and hope for the future,*

*Dr. Garry Gordon and Dr. Amy Yasko*

## Additional Suggested Resources
*for Parents and Practitioners*

Anglesey, Deborah <u>Battling the MSG Myth</u>. Front Porch Press

Blaylock, Russell L. New Developments in the Prevention and Treatment of Neurodegenerative Diseases. *JANA* 5 (2002): 15-32.

Blaylock, Russell L. <u>Excitotoxins: The Taste that Kills</u>. Sante Fe, New Mexico: Health P, 1997.

Blaylock R. The Central Role of Excitotoxicity in Autism Spectrum Disorders. *JANA* 2003; 6(1): 10.

Blaylock R. Interaction of Cytokines, Excitotoxins, and Reactive Nitrogen and Oxygen Species in Autism Spectrum Disorders. *JANA* 2003; 6(4): 21.

Gordon G. <u>The Omega-3 Miracle</u>. Freedom Press, 2004

Yasko A. The Role of Excitotoxins in Autistic Type Behavior. *www.holistichealth.com.* 2002; June 16.

Yasko A. Autism: A Twisted Tale of Virus and Thimerosal. *www.holistichealth.com.* 2003; May 31

(2) DVD Set: "Putting it All Together: An Introduction to the Multi-Factorial Approach to Autism" (available from www.longevityplus-rna.com and www.holisticheal.com)

www.gordonresearch.com
www.holistichealth.com
www.rnafoods.com
www.autismanswer.com

# Sample Detoxification Data

*"As a mother of a child who has suffered from heavy metal toxicity, I have had the privilege to work with both Dr. Amy Yasko and Dr. Garry Gordon. They have researched and developed a most effective treatment protocol for heavy metal toxicity. This treatment protocol has been profoundly effective in helping our son regain language and motor development. With deep gratitude, I endorse their commitment and work with all children who have developmental and neurological problems."*

Elizabeth S.

## URINE TOXIC METALS

LAB#:
PATIENT:
SEX: Male
AGE: 7

CLIENT#: 27080
DOCTOR: Amy Yasko, ND
Holistic Health
Po Box 309
Bethel, ME 04217

### POTENTIALLY TOXIC METALS

| METALS | RESULT µg/g CREAT | REFERENCE RANGE | | WITHIN REFERENCE RANGE | ELEVATED | VERY ELEVATED |
|---|---|---|---|---|---|---|
| Aluminum | < dl | < | 60 | | | |
| Antimony | < dl | < | 1.5 | | | |
| Arsenic | 35 | < | 130 | | | |
| Beryllium | < dl | < | 0.6 | | | |
| Bismuth | < dl | < | 20 | | | |
| Cadmium | 21 | < | 2 | | | |
| Lead | 6.6 | < | 18 | | | |
| Mercury | < dl | < | 5 | | | |
| Nickel | 2.1 | < | 15 | | | |
| Platinum | < dl | < | 1 | | | |
| Thallium | < dl | < | 1 | | | |
| Thorium | < dl | < | 0.5 | | | |
| Tin | 0.7 | < | 15 | | | |
| Tungsten | 0.2 | < | 1.5 | | | |
| Uranium | < dl | < | 0.2 | | | |

### CREATININE

| | RESULT mg/dL | REFERENCE RANGE | 2SD LOW | 1SD LOW | MEAN | 1SD HIGH | 2SD HIGH |
|---|---|---|---|---|---|---|---|
| Creatinine | 22 | 40- 142 | | | | | |

### SPECIMEN DATA

Comments:
Date Collected: 10/18/2003
Date Received: 10/22/2003
Date Completed: 10/25/2003

Method: ICP-MS
<dl:    less than detection limit
Provoking Agent:

Collection Period: **timed: 3 hours**
Volume:
Provocation:

# URINE TOXIC METALS

LAB#:
PATIENT:
SEX: Male
AGE: 4

CLIENT#: 27080
DOCTOR: Amy Yasko, ND
Holistic Health
Po Box 309
Bethel, ME 04217

## POTENTIALLY TOXIC METALS

| METALS | RESULT µg/g CREAT | REFERENCE RANGE | WITHIN REFERENCE RANGE | ELEVATED | VERY ELEVATED |
|---|---|---|---|---|---|
| Aluminum | < dl | < 35 | | | |
| Antimony | < dl | < 5 | | | |
| Arsenic | 92 | < 100 | ▬▬▬▬▬▬▬ | | |
| Beryllium | < dl | < 0.5 | | | |
| Bismuth | < dl | < 30 | | | |
| Cadmium | < dl | < 2 | | | |
| Lead | < dl | < 15 | | | |
| Mercury | 15 | < 3 | ▬▬▬▬▬▬▬▬▬▬▬▬▬▬▬▬▬▬▬▬▬ | | |
| Nickel | < dl | < 12 | | | |
| Platinum | < dl | < 2 | | | |
| Thallium | 2.3 | < 14 | ▬▬ | | |
| Thorium | < dl | < 12 | | | |
| Tin | < dl | < 6 | | | |
| Tungsten | < dl | < 23 | | | |
| Uranium | < dl | < 1 | | | |

## CREATININE

| | RESULT mg/dL | REFERENCE RANGE | 2SD LOW   1SD LOW | MEAN | 1SD HIGH   2SD HIGH |
|---|---|---|---|---|---|
| Creatinine | 13 | 21 - 76 | ▬▬▬▬▬▬▬▬▬▬▬ | | |

## SPECIMEN DATA

Comments:
Date Collected: 8/1/2003
Date Received: 8/4/2003
Date Completed: 8/5/2003

Method: ICP-MS
<dl:   less than detection limit
Provoking Agent:

Collection Period: Random
Volume:
Provocation:   PRE PROVOCATIVE

82

# URINE TOXIC METALS

| | | |
|---|---|---|
| LAB#: | CLIENT#: 27080 | |
| PATIENT: | DOCTOR: Amy Yasko, ND | |
| SEX: Male | Holistic Health | |
| AGE: 4 | Po Box 309 | |
| | Bethel, ME 04217 | |

## POTENTIALLY TOXIC METALS

| METALS | RESULT µg/g CREAT | REFERENCE RANGE | WITHIN REFERENCE RANGE | ELEVATED | VERY ELEVATED |
|---|---|---|---|---|---|
| Aluminum | 120 | < 35 | ████████████████ | | |
| Antimony | < dl | < 5 | | | |
| Arsenic | 78 | < 100 | ████████ | | |
| Beryllium | < dl | < 0.5 | | | |
| Bismuth | < dl | < 30 | | | |
| Cadmium | 0.7 | < 2 | ███ | | |
| Lead | 3.8 | < 15 | ██ | | |
| Mercury | 12 | < 3 | ████████████████████████████ | | |
| Nickel | 5.2 | < 12 | ███ | | |
| Platinum | < dl | < 2 | | | |
| Thallium | 2.2 | < 14 | ██ | | |
| Thorium | 0.2 | < 12 | █ | | |
| Tin | 2.8 | < 6 | ████ | | |
| Tungsten | 0.3 | < 23 | █ | | |
| Uranium | < dl | < 1 | | | |

## CREATININE

| | RESULT mg/dL | REFERENCE RANGE | 2SD LOW | 1SD LOW | MEAN | 1SD HIGH | 2SD HIGH |
|---|---|---|---|---|---|---|---|
| Creatinine | 26 | 21- 76 | | ████████ | | | |

## SPECIMEN DATA

| | | | |
|---|---|---|---|
| Comments: | | | |
| Date Collected: | 8/5/2003 | Method: ICP-MS | Collection Period: Random |
| Date Received: | 8/7/2003 | <dl: less than detection limit | Volume: |
| Date Completed: | 8/15/2003 | Provoking Agent: | Provocation: POST |

83

# URINE TOXIC METALS

LAB#:
PATIENT:
SEX: Male
AGE: 4

CLIENT#: 27080
DOCTOR: Amy Yasko, ND
Holistic Health
Po Box 309
Bethel, ME 04217

## POTENTIALLY TOXIC METALS

| METALS | RESULT µg/g CREAT | REFERENCE RANGE | WITHIN REFERENCE RANGE | ELEVATED | VERY ELEVATED |
|--------|-------------------|-----------------|------------------------|----------|---------------|
| Aluminum | < dl | < 35 | | | |
| Antimony | 0.5 | < 5 | ▬ | | |
| Arsenic | 91 | < 100 | ▬▬▬▬▬▬▬▬ | | |
| Beryllium | < dl | < 0.5 | | | |
| Bismuth | < dl | < 30 | | | |
| Cadmium | 1.7 | < 2 | ▬▬▬▬▬ | | |
| Lead | < dl | < 15 | | | |
| Mercury | 19 | < 3 | ▬▬▬▬▬▬▬▬▬▬▬▬▬▬ | | |
| Nickel | 4.4 | < 12 | ▬▬▬ | | |
| Platinum | < dl | < 2 | | | |
| Thallium | 0.4 | < 14 | ▬ | | |
| Thorium | < dl | < 12 | | | |
| Tin | 1.8 | < 6 | ▬▬ | | |
| Tungsten | 5.1 | < 23 | ▬▬ | | |
| Uranium | < dl | < 1 | | | |

## CREATININE

| | RESULT mg/dL | REFERENCE RANGE | 2SD LOW | 1SD LOW | MEAN | 1SD HIGH | 2SD HIGH |
|--|--------------|-----------------|---------|---------|------|----------|----------|
| Creatinine | 14 | 21- 76 | ▬▬▬▬▬▬▬▬▬▬ | | | | |

## SPECIMEN DATA

Comments:
Date Collected: 9/13/2003   Method: ICP-MS   Collection Period: Random
Date Received: 9/15/2003   <dl:   less than detection limit   Volume:
Date Completed: 9/16/2003   Provoking Agent:   Provocation:

84

# URINE TOXIC METALS

**LAB#:**
**PATIENT:**
**SEX:** Male
**AGE:** 5

**CLIENT#:** 27080
**DOCTOR:** Amy Yasko, ND
Holistic Health
Po Box 309
Bethel, ME 04217

## POTENTIALLY TOXIC METALS

| METALS | RESULT µg/g CREAT | REFERENCE RANGE | WITHIN REFERENCE RANGE | ELEVATED | VERY ELEVATED |
|---|---|---|---|---|---|
| Aluminum | 38 | < 35 | | | |
| Antimony | < dl | < 5 | | | |
| Arsenic | 34 | < 100 | | | |
| Beryllium | < dl | < 0.5 | | | |
| Bismuth | < dl | < 30 | | | |
| Cadmium | < dl | < 2 | | | |
| Lead | 1.3 | < 15 | | | |
| Mercury | 13 | < 3 | | | |
| Nickel | 4.4 | < 12 | | | |
| Platinum | < dl | < 2 | | | |
| Thallium | 0.8 | < 14 | | | |
| Thorium | < dl | < 12 | | | |
| Tin | 2.1 | < 6 | | | |
| Tungsten | < dl | < 23 | | | |
| Uranium | < dl | < 1 | | | |

## CREATININE

| | RESULT mg/dL | REFERENCE RANGE | 2SD LOW 1SD LOW | MEAN | 1SD HIGH 2SD HIGH |
|---|---|---|---|---|---|
| Creatinine | 25 | 40- 142 | | | |

## SPECIMEN DATA

Comments:
Date Collected: 8/20/2003
Date Received: 8/22/2003
Date Completed: 8/23/2003

Method: ICP-MS
<dl: less than detection limit
Provoking Agent:

Collection Period: Random
Volume:
Provocation:

85

# URINE TOXIC METALS

LAB#:
PATIENT:
SEX: Male
AGE: 4

CLIENT#: 27080
DOCTOR: Amy Yasko, ND
Holistic Health
Po Box 309
Bethel, ME 04217

## POTENTIALLY TOXIC METALS

| METALS | RESULT µg/g CREAT | REFERENCE RANGE | WITHIN REFERENCE RANGE | ELEVATED | VERY ELEVATED |
|---|---|---|---|---|---|
| Aluminum | 180 | < 35 | | | |
| Antimony | 0.5 | < 5 | | | |
| Arsenic | 72 | < 100 | | | |
| Beryllium | < dl | < 0.5 | | | |
| Bismuth | < dl | < 30 | | | |
| Cadmium | 0.6 | < 2 | | | |
| Lead | < dl | < 15 | | | |
| Mercury | 10 | < 3 | | | |
| Nickel | 2.6 | < 12 | | | |
| Platinum | < dl | < 2 | | | |
| Thallium | 3.2 | < 14 | | | |
| Thorium | < dl | < 12 | | | |
| Tin | 1.2 | < 6 | | | |
| Tungsten | 3.5 | < 23 | | | |
| Uranium | < dl | < 1 | | | |

## CREATININE

| | RESULT mg/dL | REFERENCE RANGE | 2SD LOW | 1SD LOW | MEAN | 1SD HIGH | 2SD HIGH |
|---|---|---|---|---|---|---|---|
| Creatinine | 14 | 21- 76 | | | | | |

## SPECIMEN DATA

Comments:
Date Collected: 7/24/2003
Date Received: 7/25/2003
Date Completed: 7/29/2003

Method: ICP-MS
<dl: less than detection limit
Provoking Agent:

Collection Period: Random
Volume:
Provocation: PRE PROVOCATIVE

86

# URINE TOXIC METALS

**LAB#:**
**PATIENT:**
**SEX:** Male
**AGE:** 3

**CLIENT#:** 27080
**DOCTOR:** Amy Yasko, ND
Holistic Health
Po Box 309
Bethel, ME 04217

## POTENTIALLY TOXIC METALS

| METALS | RESULT µg/g CREAT | REFERENCE RANGE | WITHIN REFERENCE RANGE | ELEVATED | VERY ELEVATED |
|---|---|---|---|---|---|
| Aluminum | 40 | < 35 | ████████████ | | |
| Antimony | 0.2 | < 5 | █ | | |
| Arsenic | 23 | < 100 | ██ | | |
| Beryllium | < dl | < 0.5 | | | |
| Bismuth | < dl | < 30 | | | |
| Cadmium | 0.7 | < 2 | ██ | | |
| Lead | 16 | < 15 | █████████ | | |
| Mercury | 1.7 | < 3 | █████ | | |
| Nickel | 2.2 | < 12 | ██ | | |
| Platinum | < dl | < 2 | | | |
| Thallium | 0.8 | < 14 | █ | | |
| Thorium | < dl | < 12 | | | |
| Tin | 97 | < 6 | ████████████████████████████████ | | |
| Tungsten | 0.2 | < 23 | █ | | |
| Uranium | < dl | < 1 | | | |

## CREATININE

| | RESULT mg/dL | REFERENCE RANGE | 2SD LOW | 1SD LOW | MEAN | 1SD HIGH | 2SD HIGH |
|---|---|---|---|---|---|---|---|
| Creatinine | 45 | 21 - 76 | | | ██ | | |

## SPECIMEN DATA

Comments:
Date Collected: 9/17/2003       Method: ICP-MS                 Collection Period: Random
Date Received: 9/19/2003        <dl:  less than detection limit   Volume:
Date Completed: 9/20/2003       Provoking Agent:               Provocation:

87

# URINE TOXIC METALS

LAB#:
PATIENT:
SEX: Male
AGE: 3

CLIENT#: 27080
DOCTOR: Amy Yasko, ND
Holistic Health
Po Box 309
Bethel, ME 04217

## POTENTIALLY TOXIC METALS

| METALS | RESULT µg/g CREAT | REFERENCE RANGE | WITHIN REFERENCE RANGE | ELEVATED | VERY ELEVATED |
|---|---|---|---|---|---|
| Aluminum | 82 | < 35 | | | |
| Antimony | 0.3 | < 5 | | | |
| Arsenic | 14 | < 100 | | | |
| Beryllium | < dl | < 0.5 | | | |
| Bismuth | 0.3 | < 30 | | | |
| Cadmium | 5.5 | < 2 | | | |
| Lead | 5.4 | < 15 | | | |
| Mercury | < dl | < 3 | | | |
| Nickel | 5.3 | < 12 | | | |
| Platinum | < dl | < 2 | | | |
| Thallium | 0.5 | < 14 | | | |
| Thorium | 0.07 | < 12 | | | |
| Tin | 140 | < 6 | | | |
| Tungsten | 0.1 | < 23 | | | |
| Uranium | 0.1 | < 1 | | | |

## CREATININE

| | RESULT mg/dL | REFERENCE RANGE | 2SD LOW | 1SD LOW | MEAN | 1SD HIGH | 2SD HIGH |
|---|---|---|---|---|---|---|---|
| Creatinine | 37 | 21- 76 | | | | | |

## SPECIMEN DATA

Comments: **results checked**
Date Collected: 9/19/2003
Date Received: 9/22/2003
Date Completed: 9/24/2003

Method: **ICP-MS**
<dl: **less than detection limit**
Provoking Agent:

Collection Period: **Random**
Volume:
Provocation:

88

# URINE TOXIC METALS

**LAB#:**
**PATIENT:**
**SEX:** Male
**AGE:** 7

**CLIENT#:** 27080
**DOCTOR:** Amy Yasko, ND
Holistic Health
Po Box 309
Bethel, ME 04217

## POTENTIALLY TOXIC METALS

| METALS | RESULT µg/g CREAT | REFERENCE RANGE | WITHIN REFERENCE RANGE | ELEVATED | VERY ELEVATED |
|---|---|---|---|---|---|
| Aluminum | < dl | < 60 | | | |
| Antimony | < dl | < 1.5 | | | |
| Arsenic | 54 | < 130 | ▬▬▬ | | |
| Beryllium | < dl | < 0.6 | | | |
| Bismuth | < dl | < 20 | | | |
| Cadmium | 0.7 | < 2 | ▬▬▬ | | |
| Lead | < dl | < 18 | | | |
| Mercury | 1.1 | < 5 | ▬ | | |
| Nickel | 4.8 | < 15 | ▬▬ | | |
| Platinum | < dl | < 1 | | | |
| Thallium | < dl | < 1 | | | |
| Thorium | < dl | < 0.5 | | | |
| Tin | < dl | < 15 | | | |
| Tungsten | 5.7 | < 1.5 | ▬▬▬▬▬▬▬▬▬ | | |
| Uranium | < dl | < 0.2 | | | |

## CREATININE

| | RESULT mg/dL | REFERENCE RANGE | 2SD LOW  1SD LOW | MEAN | 1SD HIGH   2SD HIGH |
|---|---|---|---|---|---|
| Creatinine | 55 | 40- 142 | | ▬▬▬▬▬ | |

## SPECIMEN DATA

Comments:
Date Collected: 10/14/2003
Date Received: 10/16/2003
Date Completed: 10/23/2003

Method: ICP-MS
<dl: less than detection limit
Provoking Agent:

Collection Period: timed: 2 hours
Volume:
Provocation: POST PROVOCATIVE

89

# URINE TOXIC METALS

| | | |
|---|---|---|
| **LAB#:** | **CLIENT#:** 27080 | |
| **PATIENT:** | **DOCTOR:** Amy Yasko, ND | |
| **SEX:** Male | Holistic Health | |
| **AGE:** 4 | Po Box 309 | |
| | Bethel, ME 04217 | |

## POTENTIALLY TOXIC METALS

| METALS | RESULT µg/g CREAT | REFERENCE RANGE | WITHIN REFERENCE RANGE | ELEVATED | VERY ELEVATED |
|---|---|---|---|---|---|
| Aluminum | < dl | < 35 | | | |
| Antimony | < dl | < 5 | | | |
| Arsenic | 38 | < 100 | ▬ | | |
| Beryllium | < dl | < 0.5 | | | |
| Bismuth | < dl | < 30 | | | |
| Cadmium | < dl | < 2 | | | |
| Lead | 33 | < 15 | ▬▬▬▬▬ | | |
| Mercury | 24 | < 3 | ▬▬▬▬▬▬▬▬▬▬▬ | | |
| Nickel | < dl | < 12 | | | |
| Platinum | < dl | < 2 | | | |
| Thallium | < dl | < 14 | | | |
| Thorium | < dl | < 12 | | | |
| Tin | < dl | < 6 | | | |
| Tungsten | < dl | < 23 | | | |
| Uranium | < dl | < 1 | | | |

## CREATININE

| | RESULT mg/dL | REFERENCE RANGE | 2SD LOW | 1SD LOW | MEAN | 1SD HIGH | 2SD HIGH |
|---|---|---|---|---|---|---|---|
| Creatinine | 4.6 | 21 - 76 | ▬▬▬▬▬▬▬▬ | | | | |

## SPECIMEN DATA

Comments:

| | | | | | |
|---|---|---|---|---|---|
| Date Collected: | 8/21/2003 | Method: ICP-MS | | Collection Period: | Random |
| Date Received: | 8/22/2003 | <dl: less than detection limit | | Volume: | |
| Date Completed: | 8/23/2003 | Provoking Agent: | | Provocation: | PRE PROVOCATIVE |

# URINE TOXIC METALS

LAB#:
PATIENT:
SEX: Male
AGE: 7

CLIENT#: 27080
DOCTOR: Amy Yasko, ND
Holistic Health
Po Box 309
Bethel, ME 04217

## POTENTIALLY TOXIC METALS

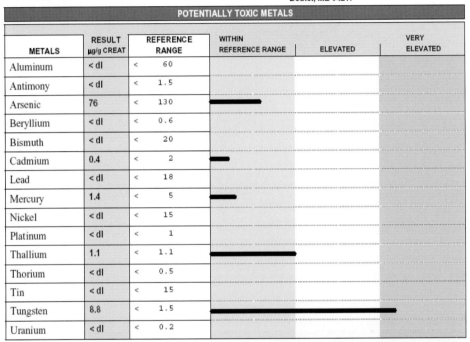

| METALS | RESULT µg/g CREAT | REFERENCE RANGE | WITHIN REFERENCE RANGE | ELEVATED | VERY ELEVATED |
|---|---|---|---|---|---|
| Aluminum | < dl | < 60 | | | |
| Antimony | < dl | < 1.5 | | | |
| Arsenic | 76 | < 130 | | | |
| Beryllium | < dl | < 0.6 | | | |
| Bismuth | < dl | < 20 | | | |
| Cadmium | 0.4 | < 2 | | | |
| Lead | < dl | < 18 | | | |
| Mercury | 1.4 | < 5 | | | |
| Nickel | < dl | < 15 | | | |
| Platinum | < dl | < 1 | | | |
| Thallium | 1.1 | < 1.1 | | | |
| Thorium | < dl | < 0.5 | | | |
| Tin | < dl | < 15 | | | |
| Tungsten | 8.8 | < 1.5 | | | |
| Uranium | < dl | < 0.2 | | | |

## CREATININE

| | RESULT mg/dL | REFERENCE RANGE | 2SD LOW  1SD LOW | MEAN | 1SD HIGH  2SD HIGH |
|---|---|---|---|---|---|
| Creatinine | 30 | 40- 142 | | | |

## SPECIMEN DATA

Comments:
Date Collected: 11/3/2003
Date Received: 11/4/2003
Date Completed: 11/10/2003

Method: ICP-MS
<dl: less than detection limit
Provoking Agent:

Collection Period: Random
Volume:
Provocation: POST PROVOCATIVE

# URINE TOXIC METALS

| | | |
|---|---|---|
| **LAB#:** | **CLIENT#:** 27080 | |
| **PATIENT:** | **DOCTOR:** Amy Yasko, ND | |
| **SEX:** Male | Holistic Health | |
| **AGE:** 8 | Po Box 309 | |
| | Bethel, ME 04217 | |

## POTENTIALLY TOXIC METALS

| METALS | RESULT µg/g CREAT | REFERENCE RANGE | WITHIN REFERENCE RANGE | ELEVATED | VERY ELEVATED |
|---|---|---|---|---|---|
| Aluminum | < dl | < 60 | | | |
| Antimony | < dl | < 1.5 | | | |
| Arsenic | 17 | < 130 | ▬ | | |
| Beryllium | < dl | < 0.6 | | | |
| Bismuth | < dl | < 20 | | | |
| Cadmium | < dl | < 2 | | | |
| Lead | 2.1 | < 18 | ▬ | | |
| Mercury | 12 | < 5 | ▬▬▬▬▬▬▬▬ | | |
| Nickel | < dl | < 15 | | | |
| Platinum | < dl | < 1 | | | |
| Thallium | < dl | < 1.1 | | | |
| Thorium | < dl | < 0.5 | | | |
| Tin | < dl | < 15 | | | |
| Tungsten | 0.7 | < 1.5 | ▬▬ | | |
| Uranium | < dl | < 0.2 | | | |

## CREATININE

| | RESULT mg/dL | REFERENCE RANGE | 2SD LOW 1SD LOW | MEAN | 1SD HIGH 2SD HIGH |
|---|---|---|---|---|---|
| Creatinine | 8.2 | 40 - 142 | ▬▬▬▬▬▬▬ | | |

## SPECIMEN DATA

Comments:

| | | | |
|---|---|---|---|
| Date Collected: | 11/18/2003 | Method: ICP-MS | Collection Period: Random |
| Date Received: | 11/19/2003 | <dl: less than detection limit | Volume: |
| Date Completed: | 11/20/2003 | Provoking Agent: | Provocation: PRE PROVOCATIVE |

# URINE TOXIC METALS

**LAB#:**
**PATIENT:**
**SEX:** Male
**AGE:** 8

**CLIENT#:** 27080
**DOCTOR:** Amy Yasko, ND
Holistic Health
Po Box 309
Bethel, ME 04217

## POTENTIALLY TOXIC METALS

| METALS | RESULT µg/g CREAT | REFERENCE RANGE | WITHIN REFERENCE RANGE | ELEVATED | VERY ELEVATED |
|--------|--------|--------|--------|--------|--------|
| Aluminum | < dl | < 60 | | | |
| Antimony | < dl | < 1.5 | | | |
| Arsenic | 37 | < 130 | ▬▬ | | |
| Beryllium | < dl | < 0.6 | | | |
| Bismuth | < dl | < 20 | | | |
| Cadmium | < dl | < 2 | | | |
| Lead | < dl | < 18 | | | |
| Mercury | 12 | < 5 | ▬▬▬▬▬▬▬▬▬ | | |
| Nickel | < dl | < 15 | | | |
| Platinum | < dl | < 1 | | | |
| Thallium | 0.5 | < 1.1 | ▬▬▬ | | |
| Thorium | < dl | < 0.5 | | | |
| Tin | < dl | < 15 | | | |
| Tungsten | < dl | < 1.5 | | | |
| Uranium | < dl | < 0.2 | | | |

## CREATININE

| | RESULT mg/dL | REFERENCE RANGE | 2SD LOW | 1SD LOW | MEAN | 1SD HIGH | 2SD HIGH |
|--|--|--|--|--|--|--|--|
| Creatinine | 15 | 40- 142 | ▬▬▬▬▬▬▬▬ | | | | |

## SPECIMEN DATA

Comments:
Date Collected: 2/24/2004   Method: ICP-MS   Collection Period: Random
Date Received: 2/26/2004   <dl:  less than detection limit   Volume:
Date Completed: 2/28/2004   Provoking Agent:   Provocation: POST PROVOCATIVF

93

# URINE TOXIC METALS

LAB#:
PATIENT:
SEX: Male
AGE: 6

CLIENT#: 27080
DOCTOR: Amy Yasko, ND
Holistic Health
Po Box 309
Bethel, ME 04217

## POTENTIALLY TOXIC METALS

| METALS | RESULT µg/g CREAT | REFERENCE RANGE | WITHIN REFERENCE RANGE | ELEVATED | VERY ELEVATED |
|---|---|---|---|---|---|
| Aluminum | < dl | < 60 | | | |
| Antimony | < dl | < 1.5 | | | |
| Arsenic | 47 | < 130 | ▬▬ | | |
| Beryllium | < dl | < 0.6 | | | |
| Bismuth | < dl | < 20 | | | |
| Cadmium | 0.8 | < 2 | ▬▬ | | |
| Lead | < dl | < 18 | | | |
| Mercury | 11 | < 5 | ▬▬▬▬▬▬▬▬ | | |
| Nickel | < dl | < 15 | | | |
| Platinum | < dl | < 1 | | | |
| Thallium | 1.2 | < 1.1 | ▬▬▬▬▬ | | |
| Thorium | < dl | < 0.5 | | | |
| Tin | < dl | < 15 | | | |
| Tungsten | < dl | < 1.5 | | | |
| Uranium | < dl | < 0.2 | | | |

## CREATININE

| | RESULT mg/dL | REFERENCE RANGE | 2SD LOW | 1SD LOW | MEAN | 1SD HIGH | 2SD HIGH |
|---|---|---|---|---|---|---|---|
| Creatinine | 11 | 40- 142 | ▬▬▬▬▬▬▬▬ | | | | |

## SPECIMEN DATA

Comments:
Date Collected: 3/18/2004
Date Received: 3/24/2004
Date Completed: 3/25/2004

Method: ICP-MS
<dl: less than detection limit
Provoking Agent:

Collection Period: Random
Volume:
Provocation:

94

# URINE TOXIC METALS

**LAB#:**
**PATIENT:**
**SEX:** Male
**AGE:** 3

**CLIENT#:** 27080
**DOCTOR:** Amy Yasko, ND
Holistic Health
Po Box 309
Bethel, ME 04217

## POTENTIALLY TOXIC METALS

| METALS | RESULT µg/g CREAT | REFERENCE RANGE | WITHIN REFERENCE RANGE | ELEVATED | VERY ELEVATED |
|--------|-------------------|-----------------|------------------------|----------|---------------|
| Aluminum | < dl | < 100 | | | |
| Antimony | < dl | < 2 | | | |
| Arsenic | 140 | < 200 | ▬▬▬▬ | | |
| Beryllium | < dl | < 0.6 | | | |
| Bismuth | < dl | < 20 | | | |
| Cadmium | 7.9 | < 3 | ▬▬▬▬▬▬▬▬▬▬▬▬▬ | | |
| Lead | 0.4 | < 20 | ▬ | | |
| Mercury | 1.5 | < 5 | ▬▬ | | |
| Nickel | 7.5 | < 20 | ▬▬ | | |
| Platinum | < dl | < 1 | | | |
| Thallium | 0.2 | < 1.1 | ▬ | | |
| Thorium | < dl | < 1 | | | |
| Tin | 11 | < 20 | ▬▬▬ | | |
| Tungsten | 0.6 | < 2 | ▬▬ | | |
| Uranium | < dl | < 0.3 | | | |

## CREATININE

| | RESULT mg/dL | REFERENCE RANGE | 2SD LOW | 1SD LOW | MEAN | 1SD HIGH | 2SD HIGH |
|--|--------------|-----------------|---------|---------|------|----------|----------|
| Creatinine | 45 | 21 - 76 | | | ▬ | | |

## SPECIMEN DATA

Comments:
Date Collected: 3/30/2004
Date Received: 4/1/2004
Date Completed: 4/2/2004

Method: ICP-MS
<dl: less than detection limit
Provoking Agent:

Collection Period: Random
Volume:
Provocation:

95

# URINE TOXIC METALS

LAB#:
PATIENT:
SEX: Male
AGE: 6

CLIENT#: 27080
DOCTOR: Amy Yasko, ND
Holistic Health
Po Box 309
Bethel, ME 04217

## POTENTIALLY TOXIC METALS

| METALS | RESULT µg/g CREAT | REFERENCE RANGE | WITHIN REFERENCE RANGE | ELEVATED | VERY ELEVATED |
|---|---|---|---|---|---|
| Aluminum | < dl | < 60 | | | |
| Antimony | < dl | < 1.5 | | | |
| Arsenic | 38 | < 130 | ▬▬ | | |
| Beryllium | < dl | < 0.6 | | | |
| Bismuth | < dl | < 20 | | | |
| Cadmium | < dl | < 2 | | | |
| Lead | < dl | < 18 | | | |
| Mercury | 10 | < 5 | ▬▬▬▬▬▬ | | |
| Nickel | < dl | < 15 | | | |
| Platinum | < dl | < 1 | | | |
| Thallium | 0.7 | < 1.1 | ▬▬▬ | | |
| Thorium | < dl | < 0.5 | | | |
| Tin | < dl | < 15 | | | |
| Tungsten | < dl | < 1.5 | | | |
| Uranium | < dl | < 0.2 | | | |

## CREATININE

| | RESULT mg/dL | REFERENCE RANGE | 2SD LOW  1SD LOW | MEAN | 1SD HIGH  2SD HIGH |
|---|---|---|---|---|---|
| Creatinine | 14 | 40- 142 | ▬▬▬▬▬▬▬ | | |

## SPECIMEN DATA

Comments:
Date Collected: 3/23/2004      Method: ICP-MS              Collection Period: Random
Date Received: 3/31/2004       <dl:    less than detection limit    Volume:
Date Completed: 4/1/2004       Provoking Agent:            Provocation:

96

# URINE TOXIC METALS

LAB#:
PATIENT:
SEX: Male
AGE: 4

CLIENT#: 27080
DOCTOR: Amy Yasko, ND
Holistic Health
Po Box 309
Bethel, ME 04217

## POTENTIALLY TOXIC METALS

| METALS | RESULT µg/g CREAT | REFERENCE RANGE | WITHIN REFERENCE RANGE | ELEVATED | VERY ELEVATED |
|---|---|---|---|---|---|
| Aluminum | < dl | < 35 | | | |
| Antimony | < dl | < 5 | | | |
| Arsenic | 58 | < 100 | | | |
| Beryllium | < dl | < 0.5 | | | |
| Bismuth | 0.4 | < 30 | | | |
| Cadmium | 0.4 | < 2 | | | |
| Lead | < dl | < 15 | | | |
| Mercury | 6.8 | < 3 | | | |
| Nickel | < dl | < 12 | | | |
| Platinum | < dl | < 2 | | | |
| Thallium | 0.3 | < 14 | | | |
| Thorium | 0.1 | < 12 | | | |
| Tin | 1.4 | < 6 | | | |
| Tungsten | 0.4 | < 23 | | | |
| Uranium | 0.1 | < 1 | | | |

## CREATININE

| | RESULT mg/dL | REFERENCE RANGE | 2SD LOW  1SD LOW | MEAN | 1SD HIGH  2SD HIGH |
|---|---|---|---|---|---|
| Creatinine | 23 | 21- 76 | | | |

## SPECIMEN DATA

Comments:
Date Collected: 9/20/2003
Date Received: 9/22/2003
Date Completed: 9/24/2003

Method: ICP-MS
<dl:    less than detection limit
Provoking Agent:

Collection Period: Random
Volume:
Provocation:

97

# FECAL METALS

| LAB# | | CLIENT#: 27080 |
|---|---|---|
| PATIENT: | | DOCTOR: Amy Yasko, ND |
| SEX: Male | | Holistic Health |
| AGE: 4 | | Po Box 309 |
| | | Bethel, ME 04217 |

## POTENTIALLY TOXIC METALS

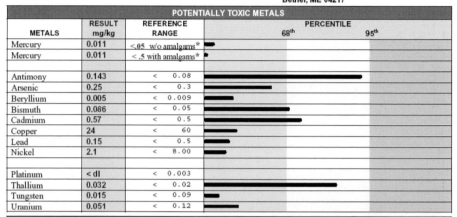

| METALS | RESULT mg/kg | REFERENCE RANGE | PERCENTILE 68th | 95th |
|---|---|---|---|---|
| Mercury | 0.011 | <.05 w/o amalgams* | | |
| Mercury | 0.011 | < .5 with amalgams* | | |
| | | | | |
| Antimony | 0.143 | < 0.08 | | |
| Arsenic | 0.25 | < 0.3 | | |
| Beryllium | 0.005 | < 0.009 | | |
| Bismuth | 0.086 | < 0.05 | | |
| Cadmium | 0.57 | < 0.5 | | |
| Copper | 24 | < 60 | | |
| Lead | 0.15 | < 0.5 | | |
| Nickel | 2.1 | < 8.00 | | |
| | | | | |
| Platinum | < dl | < 0.003 | | |
| Thallium | 0.032 | < 0.02 | | |
| Tungsten | 0.015 | < 0.09 | | |
| Uranium | 0.051 | < 0.12 | | |

## % WATER CONTENT

| | RESULT % H₂O | EXPECTED RANGE | 2SD LOW | 1SD LOW | MEAN 72.5% | 1SD HIGH | 2SD HIGH |
|---|---|---|---|---|---|---|---|
| % WATER CONTENT | 84.7 | 60-85% | | | | | |

# FECAL METALS

| LAB#: | | CLIENT#: 27080 |
|---|---|---|
| PATIENT: | | DOCTOR: Amy Yasko, ND |
| SEX: Male | | Holistic Health |
| AGE: 8 | | Po Box 309 |
| | | Bethel, ME 04217 |

## POTENTIALLY TOXIC METALS

| METALS | RESULT mg/kg | REFERENCE RANGE | PERCENTILE 68th | 95th |
|---|---|---|---|---|
| Mercury | 0.158 | <.05 w/o amalgams* | | |
| Mercury | 0.158 | < .5 with amalgams* | | |
| | | | | |
| Antimony | 0.026 | < 0.080 | | |
| Arsenic | 0.09 | < 0.30 | | |
| Beryllium | < dl | < 0.009 | | |
| Bismuth | 0.008 | < 0.050 | | |
| Cadmium | 0.02 | < 0.50 | | |
| Copper | 8 | < 60 | | |
| Lead | 0.17 | < 0.50 | | |
| Nickel | 0.7 | < 8.0 | | |
| | | | | |
| Platinum | 0.003 | < 0.003 | | |
| Thallium | < dl | < 0.020 | | |
| Tungsten | 0.018 | < 0.090 | | |
| Uranium | 0.088 | < 0.120 | | |

## % WATER CONTENT

| | RESULT % H₂O | EXPECTED RANGE | 2SD LOW | 1SD LOW | MEAN 72.5% | 1SD HIGH | 2SD HIGH |
|---|---|---|---|---|---|---|---|
| % WATER CONTENT | 98.2 | 60-85% | | | | | |

# FECAL METALS

LAB#: |
PATIENT:
SEX: Male
AGE: 8

CLIENT#: 27080
DOCTOR: Amy Yasko, ND
Holistic Health
Po Box 309
Bethel, ME 04217

## POTENTIALLY TOXIC METALS

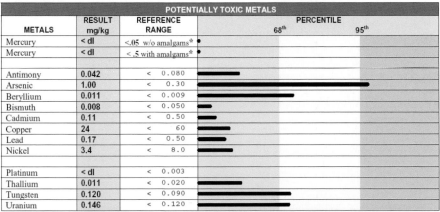

| METALS | RESULT mg/kg | REFERENCE RANGE | PERCENTILE 68th | 95th |
|---|---|---|---|---|
| Mercury | < dl | <.05 w/o amalgams* | | |
| Mercury | < dl | < .5 with amalgams* | | |
| Antimony | 0.042 | < 0.080 | | |
| Arsenic | 1.00 | < 0.30 | | |
| Beryllium | 0.011 | < 0.009 | | |
| Bismuth | 0.008 | < 0.050 | | |
| Cadmium | 0.11 | < 0.50 | | |
| Copper | 24 | < 60 | | |
| Lead | 0.17 | < 0.50 | | |
| Nickel | 3.4 | < 8.0 | | |
| Platinum | < dl | < 0.003 | | |
| Thallium | 0.011 | < 0.020 | | |
| Tungsten | 0.120 | < 0.090 | | |
| Uranium | 0.146 | < 0.120 | | |

## % WATER CONTENT

| | RESULT % H₂O | EXPECTED RANGE | 2SD LOW 1SD LOW | MEAN 72.5% | 1SD HIGH 2SD HIGH |
|---|---|---|---|---|---|
| % WATER CONTENT | 64 | 60-85% | | | |

---

# FECAL METALS

LAB#:
PATIENT:
SEX: Male
AGE: 4

CLIENT#: 27080
DOCTOR: Amy Yasko, ND
Holistic Health
Po Box 309
Bethel, ME 04217

## POTENTIALLY TOXIC METALS

| METALS | RESULT mg/kg | REFERENCE RANGE | PERCENTILE 68th | 95th |
|---|---|---|---|---|
| Mercury | 0.019 | <.05 w/o amalgams* | | |
| Mercury | 0.019 | < .5 with amalgams* | | |
| Antimony | 0.093 | < 0.08 | | |
| Arsenic | 0.30 | < 0.3 | | |
| Beryllium | 0.026 | < 0.009 | | |
| Bismuth | 0.052 | < 0.05 | | |
| Cadmium | 0.79 | < 0.5 | | |
| Copper | 120 | < 60 | | |
| Lead | 0.54 | < 0.5 | | |
| Nickel | 8.4 | < 8.00 | | |
| Platinum | < dl | < 0.003 | | |
| Thallium | 0.031 | < 0.02 | | |
| Tungsten | 0.044 | < 0.09 | | |
| Uranium | 0.112 | < 0.12 | | |

## % WATER CONTENT

| | RESULT % H₂O | EXPECTED RANGE | 2SD LOW 1SD LOW | MEAN 72.5% | 1SD HIGH 2SD HIGH |
|---|---|---|---|---|---|
| % WATER CONTENT | 80 | 60-85% | | | |

# FECAL METALS

LAB#:
PATIENT:
SEX: Male
AGE: 4

CLIENT#: 27080
DOCTOR: Amy Yasko, ND
Holistic Health
Po Box 309
Bethel, ME 04217

## POTENTIALLY TOXIC METALS

| METALS | RESULT mg/kg | REFERENCE RANGE | PERCENTILE 68th | 95th |
|---|---|---|---|---|
| Mercury | 0.008 | <.05 w/o amalgams* | | |
| Mercury | 0.008 | < .5 with amalgams* | | |
| | | | | |
| Antimony | 0.126 | <    0.08 | | |
| Arsenic | 0.12 | <    0.3 | | |
| Beryllium | < dl | <   0.009 | | |
| Bismuth | 0.036 | <    0.05 | | |
| Cadmium | 0.95 | <    0.5 | | |
| Copper | 40 | <     60 | | |
| Lead | 0.19 | <    0.5 | | |
| Nickel | 4.8 | <    8.00 | | |
| | | | | |
| Platinum | < dl | <   0.003 | | |
| Thallium | 0.023 | <   0.02 | | |
| Tungsten | 0.022 | <   0.09 | | |
| Uranium | 0.064 | <    0.12 | | |

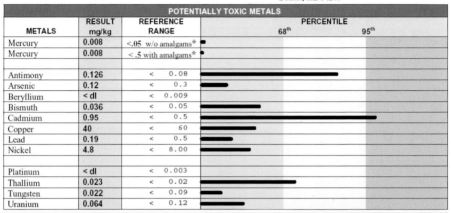

## % WATER CONTENT

| | RESULT % H₂O | EXPECTED RANGE | 2SD LOW | 1SD LOW | MEAN 72.5% | 1SD HIGH | 2SD HIGH |
|---|---|---|---|---|---|---|---|
| % WATER CONTENT | 79.4 | 60-85% | | | | | |

100

# Bibliography

A Relationship between Tylenol and Asthma.
http://illness.altmedangel.com/asthma.htm. 2002; 21 May.

Aguilar, L., et al. FgF Modifies the Brain electrical activity. *Inst. Invest.* Neuroplast. Des. Cel. 1992; August.

Aravindakumar C., et al. Nitric oxide induces Zn+ release from metallothionein by destroying zinc-sulphur clusters without concomitant formation of S-nitrosothiol. *Biochem. J.* 1999; 344:253.

Aschner, et al. Methylmercury alters glutamate transport in astrocytes. *Neurochem Int.* 2000; 37:199.

Auger, Anthony P., et al. Mechanisms Of Steroid-Induced Brain Differentiation.http://www.tmin.ac.jp/sympo/98/mccarthy.html.2002;18 Apr

Atzori, M., et al. Dopamine-Acetycholine Interactions in the Modulation of glutamate Release. *Ann N.Y. Acad. Sci.* 2003; 1003:346

Aukrust P., et al. Decreased levels of total and reduced glutathione in CD4+ lymphocytes in common variable immunodeficiencies are associated with activation of the tumor necrosis factor system: possible immunopathogenic role of oxidative stress. *Blood.* 1995; 86:1383.

Babal, P., et al. Early Postnatal Glutamate Treatment Results in Altered Vascular Responsiveness. *Endocrine Regulations* 1998; 32: 33.

Bach, JF. Regulatory T Cells Under Scrutiny. *Nature Reviews Immunology.* 2003; 3:139.

Bartlett, John G., Neil R. Blacklow, and Sherwood L. Gorbach. *Infectious Diseases.* Philadelphia, PA: W.B. Saunders Company, 1998.

Bauer A., et al. Alpha-lipoic acid is an effective inhibitor of human immunodeficiency virus (HIV-1) replication. *Klinische Wochenschrift.* 1991; 69:722.

Bayliss, M. T., and M. S. Hickery. Interleukin- induced nitric oxide inhibits sulfation of glycosaminoglycan chains. *Biochim Biophys Acta* 1998; 1425 :282.

Bernard S., et al. Autism: A Unique Type of Mercury Poisoning. www.autism.com/ari/mercurylong.html 2000; June 27.

Biello, S. M., D. A. Golombek, and M. E. Harrington. Neuropeptide Y and glutamate block phase shifts in the suprachiasmatic nucleus in vitro. http://www.psy.gla.ac.uk/people/abstract.asp 1997; 25 June 2002

Binkley, Karen. Idiopathic Environmental Intolerance. *Journal of Allergy and Clinical Immunology* 2001;107: 887.

Blaylock, Russell. Interaction of Cytokines, Excitotoxins, and Reactive Nitrogen and Oxygen Species in Autism Spectrum Disorders. *JANA* 2003; 6 (4): 21.

Blaylock R. The Central Role of Excitotoxicity in Autism Spectrum Disorders. *JANA* 2003; 6(1): 10.

Blaylock, Russell L. Phytonutrients and Metabolic Stimulants as Protection Against Neurodegeneration and Excitotoxicity. *JANA* 2000; 2: 30.

Blaylock, Russell L. New Developments in the Prevention and Treatment of Neurodegenerative Diseases. *JANA* 2002; 5: 15-32.

Blaylock, Russell L. *Excitotoxins:The Taste that Kills.* Sante Fe, New Mexico: Health P, 1997.

Blue, M. E., et al. Postmortem Brain Abnormalities of the Glutamate Neurotransmitter System in Autism. *Neurology* 2001; 57: 1618.

Brinkworth R., et al. Inhibition of HIV-1 Proteinase by Non-peptide Carboxylates. *Biochem Biophy Res Commun* 1991; 176(1):241.

Brooks, D., et al. Molecular Characterization, Reactivation, and Depletion of Latent HIV. *Immunity* 2003; 19: 413.

Buckland, J. Tolerance or Immunity-Dendritic Cells Decide. *Nature Reviews Immunology*. 2003; 3(3): 182.

Campbell, J., M. A. Drake, and J. H. Isonhood. Impact of Salt and MSG on Survival of E. coli.
http://ift.confex.com/ift/2002/techprogram/paper_13227.htm. 2002; 17 June

Carboxylation of glutamic acid. *The Merck Manual* (n.d.). 8 May 2002
http://www.merck.com/pubs/mmanual/figures/3fig2.htm.

Carlos, Juan. A New Look at Lipids in Nerves. *Nature Reviews*, 2004; 5.

Chelation of Mercury for the Treatment of Autism. 3 Mar. 2002
http://www.healing-arts.org/children/holmes.htm.

Clarkson T. The Three Modern Faces of Mercury. *Environmental Health Perspectives*. 2002; 110:11.

Cleary, P. P., Gary M. Dunny, and Larry L. McKay. Genetics *and Molecular Biology of Streptococci, Lactococci, and Enterococci.*
Washington, DC: American Society for Microbiology, 1999.

Correll, et al. Use of Chemically Modified Nucleotides to Determine a 62 Nucleotide RNA Crystal Structure: A Survey of Phosphorothioates, Br, Pt, & Hg. *J Biomolecular Structure and Dynamics* 1997; 15(2):165

D'Adamo, Peter, and Catherine Whitney. *Eat Right 4 Your Type*. New York, NY: G.P. Putnam's Sons, 1996.

Daniels, Daniel H., Gregory W. Diachenko, and Frank L. Joe, Jr. Determination of Free Glutamic Acid in a Variety of Foods by High-performance Liquid Chromatography. *Food Additives and Contaminants* 1995;12 : 21-29.

Demirham I., Inhibition of Tat-mediated HIV-1-LTR Transactivation and Virus Replication by Sulfhydryl Compounds with Chelating Properties. *Anticancer Res.* 2000 ;20(4):2515.

Deth, Richard. Molecular *Origins of Human Attention, The Dopamine-Folate Connection*. Published by Kluwer.

Disease Statistics. http://www.msgtruth.org/disease.htm.9 June 2002

Drugs tested for Lou Gehrig's disease. *Science News* 2001; 160:23.

Dube, G. R., et al. Genetic enhancement of learning and memory in mice. *Nature* 1999; 401:63.

Edwards, C., et al. Auditory Midbrain Neurons That Count. *Nature Neuroscience* 2002; 5(10):934.

Effect Of Altered Expression Of The Cytoplasmic Copper-Zinc Superoxide Dismutase On Oxidative Stress Mediated Phenomena. http://lanfiles.williams.edu/~eadler/thesis/PJS1.html 1997; 25 June 2002.

Effects of Estrogens on Erythrocyte Antioxidant Superoxide Dismutase, Catalase and Glutathione Peroxidase Activities During Menstrual Cycle. *J Endocrinology* 2000; 167(3):447.

Eisenberg, J., et al. Haplotype Relative Risk Study of COMT and ADHD: Association of the High-enzyme Activity. *Am J. Med. Genet.* 1999; 88(5):497.

Evolutionary Discordance of Grains/Legumes in Diet. http://grains-legumes-b. html 18 June 2002.

Explorations of the New Frontier between Gut and Brain: A look at GAGs, CCK and Motilin. *1998 Durham Conference Psychobiology of Autism* http:// sunderland.ac.uk/autism.1998; 7 May 2002

Fleming, Richard and Tom Monte. *Stop Inflammation Now!* 2004

Florance, C. *Maverick Mind.* Published G.P. Putnam's Sons New York 2003.

Focus on Music. *Nature Neuroscience* 2003; 6(7) July.

Folkerth, Rebecca D., Preliminary Evidence: Herpesvirus Link to Mesial Temporal Lobe Epilepsy. *Jour. Watch Neur.* 2004; 6(3): 20.

From Inflammation and Autoimmunity to Nerve Regeneration and Protection. http://www.sciencedaily.com. 1999

Fujinami, R. and T. Sweeten. Letting Antibodies Get to Your Head. *Nature Medicine* 2003; 9(7):823.

Funseth E., et al. Effects of Coxsackievirus B3 Infection on Acute-phase Protein Metallothionein and on Cytochrome P-4501A1. *Sci Total Environ* 2002; 284(1):37.

Geiss G., et al. Global Impact of Influenza Virus on Cellular Pathways Is Mediated by Both Replication-Dependent and Independent Events. *J Virology* 2001; 75(9):4321.

Giacometti, T. Free and Bound Glutamate in Natural Products. Glutamic Acid:Advances in *Biochemistry and Physiology* 1979.

Glutamine: The Essential 'Non-Essential' Amino Acid. *Life Extension Magazine* 2002;199.

Gordon, G. EDTA and Chelation Therapy: History and Mechanisms of Action An Update. *Clinical Practice of Alternative Medicine* 2001; Volume 2(1):36-45.

Gordon, G. CHELATION DOCTOR, ASK YOURSELF "WHAT IF?" A Response to April Update by Elmer Cranton. *ACAM Journal* June 2003.

Gordon, G. and Joiner-Bey, H. *The Omega-3 Miracle.* 2004. Published by Freedom Press.

Gordon, G. and Yasko, A. Are RNA-Based Therapies the Biggest Breakthrough in NUTRITIONAL and Molecular Medicine? *Explore* 2004; 13(2):33-37.

Gould, S., et al. The Trojan Exosome Hypothesis. *PNAS* 2003; 100(19):10592.

Hans D., et al. Protection Against Glutamate-induced Cytotoxicity in C6 Glial Cells by Thiol Antioxidants. *Am J. Physiol* 1997; 273:1771.

Harder, B. Target: Celiac Disease. *Science News* . 2003; 163:392.

Hafez M., et al Susceptibility to Over Production of Cytokines in Acute Rheumatic Carditis and Their Role in the Pathogenesis. *J. Med. Sci.* 2002; 2(2):65.

Herbert, M. R. Localization of white matter volume increase in autism and developmental language disorder. *Annals of Neurology* 2004; 55:530.

Herman, J.G. and Baylin, S. Gene Silencing in Cancer in Association with Promoter Hypermethyation. *N. Engl J Med* 2003; 349:2042.

Hickery, M.S. and M.T. Bayliss. Interleukin- induced Nitric Oxide Inhibits Sulfation of Glycosaminoglycan Chains. *Biochim. Biophys. Acta.*1998;1425:282.

Hoffman, K., et al. A Murine Model for Neuropsychiatric Disorders Associated with Group A Streptococcal Infection. *J Neuroscience.* 2004; 24(7):1780.

Holden, Constance. Excited by Glutamate. *Science* 2003; 300: 1866.

Holden, Constance. Zapping Memory Craving Triggers Drug Craving. *Science* 2001;292:1039.

Hood, Ernie. RNAi: What's All the Noise About Gene Silencing? *Environmental Health Perspectives.* 2004; 112(4):A225-A229.

Ilback N., et al. Effects of Methylmercury on Cytokines, Inflammation, and Virus Clearance in a Common Infection. *Toxicology Letters* 1996; 89(1):19.

Jacoby, D. Virus-Induced Asthma Attacks. *J American Medical Association.* 2002. Vol 287:755.

Jacoby, M. Magnetic Fields and Unpolarized Light Have Hand in Chirality. *C & En.* 2000; 26:14.

Jezova, D., and D. Tokarev. Effect of Nitric Oxide Inhibition on Blood Pressure. *Physiol. Res.* 2000; 49:S87.

Jonata, P., et al. The Cortical Topography of Tonal Structures Underlying Western Music. *Science.* 2002; 298:2167.

Kasuya, E., et al. An increase in Glutamate Release in Female Rhesus Monkeys. *J. Neuroendocrinol.* 1999; 11:275.

Kasuya E., et al. A Role of GABA and Glutamate in Control of Puberty in Female. Rhesus Monkeys. *Endocrinology* 1999; 140(2):705.

Kegak, B. In Vitro Determaination of Specific Toxicity in Tetanus Vaccines. *Dev. Biol.* 2002; 111:27.

Kerblat, I. Tetanus Toxin L Chain is Processed by MHC Class I and Class II. *Immunology* 2000; 100:178.

Koland J. *Antineoplastic Agents I & II.* 2003; www.medicine.uiowa.edu/pharmacology/Lectures/ Lecturenotes/111/2004/

Lalli. G. Functional Characterization of Tentanus and Botulinum Neurotoxins Binding Domains. *J. Cell Sci.* 1999; 112:2715.

Larhammar, Dan. Neuropeptide Y and its Receptors: Physiology and Pharmacology. Molecular Properties, Ligand receptor Interactions, Roles in Appetite Regulation. 1 Dec. 2000; http://www.medfarm.neuro.uu.se/larhammar.html

Larson, H. Virtual Lab Conference. *Proceedings of the Fourth Session.* March 1-31 2003. www.afibbers.org/conference

Lee, T. H., et al. The role of Insulin in Interaction of Secretin and Cholecystokinin. *Pancreas* 12 (1996): 58.

Leo, M. A., and C. S. Lieber. Alcohol, Vitamin A, and Beta-carotene: Adverse Interactions. *American J. Clinical Nutrition* 1999; 69:1071.

Levitt J. Anxiety and Hypoglycemia What's the Connection? *Holistic Energy Magazine*. <www.hastingspress.co.uk/hypo/levitt.htm>.

Li, B., et al. Regulation of Muscarinic Acetylcholine Function in Acetylcholinesterase Knockout Mice. *Pharmacol. Biochem. Behav*. 2003; 74:977.

Li K., et al. Cellular Response to Conditional Expression of Hepatitis C Virus Core Protein in Huh7 Cultured Human Hepatoma Cells. *Hepatology* 2002; 35(5): 1237.

Lipids and Lou Gehrig's disease. *C&EN* / 26 August 2002: 30.

Marsicano, G., et ak. CB1 Cannabinoid Receptors and On-Demand Defense Against Excitotoxicity. *Science* 2003; 302:84.

Mattson, M.P., TerryAnn Perry, and Nigel H. Greig. Learning From the Gut. *Nature Medicine*. 2003; 9(9):1113.

McMichael J., et al. The Use of Low Dose Thimerosal for the Treatment of Herpesvirus Infections Non-*Linearity Conference Belle Umass Amherst.*

Mellman, I., and B. Winckler. Neuronal Polarity: Controlling the Sorting and Diffusion of Membrane Components. *Neuron*. 1999; 23:637. Milk Proteins As Potential Diet Aids. *Life Extension Magazine* 2002; June 22.

Mogadam, Michael. *Every Heart Attack Is Preventable*. 2001

Morales, J., et al. FgF Decreases seizure Frequency and Increases GABA Uptake. *Inst. Invest. Neuroplast. Des. Cel*.1992; August.

Munro, et al. High sensitivity of mouse neuronal cells to tetanus toxin requires a GPI-anchored protein. *Biochem Biophys Res Commun*. 2001; 289(2):623.

Nubrander, Biochemical Context and Clinical Use of Methylcobalamin. http://www.autisme-montreal.com/congress/2003/Neubrander.html.

NeuroGenesis Inc. The Stress Cycle. 18 June 2002 http://www.neurogenesis.cc/stresscycle.html.

Neuropeptide Y and its receptors: physiology and pharmacology. Molecular properties, ligand receptor interactions, roles in appetite regulation; 1997 http://arbl.cvmbs.colostate.edu/hbooks/pathphys/ endocrine/bodyweight/npy.html.

Neuroprotection-Glutamate and Calpain Antagonism. 22 June 2002 http:// eardisorders.html.

Neuroscience and Music in Harmony. *New York Academy of Sciences Magazine.*2004; March.

Neyts J., et al. Effect of Iodo Deoxyuridine on Vaccinia Virus Infections in Mice. *Antimicrobial Agents and Chemotherapy* 2002; 46(9):2842.

NIAID Division of AIDS CHEMDB http://apps1.niaid.nih.gov/structsearch/ default.htm. 2003; May 7.

Nicoll, Roger A., and Rachel I. Wilson. Endocannabinoid Signaling in the Brain. *Science.* 2002; 296 :678.

Nitrogen Metabolism and the Urea Cycle. 21 June 2002 http://216.23.../nitrogen-metabolism.html.

Nucleotides. www.rpi.edu/dept/bcbp/molbiochem/BiochSci/sbello/ molbioch/nucleotides.htm.

Parslow, Tristram G., Daniel P. Stites, and Abba I. Terr. *Medical Immunology.* Stamford, CT: Appleton & Lange, 1997.

Poland, G., et al. The Association Between Measles Vaccine-induced Antibody Response and the HLA-DQA1 Alleles. *Vaccines 97,* page 229 Cold Spring Harbor Press.

Purcell, A.E., Jeon, O.H., Zimmerman, A.W., Blue, M.E, Pevsner, J. Postmortem Brain Abnormalities of the Glutamate Neurotransmitter System in Autism. *Neurology* 2001; 57(9): 1618-28.

Raloff, J. Little Vessels React to Magnetic Switch. *Science News* 2003; 163:270.

Scallet, A. C. Excitotoxic Mechanisms of Neurodegeneration in Transmissible Spongiform Encephalopathies. *Ann N Y Acad Sci.* 1997;Oct.

Schoonenberg, T. In the Blink of an Eye. Movement Disorders Team Report. www.hapsonline.org/public_http/Articles/EyeTroubles.pdf.

Seppa, Nathan. Glutamate Glut Linked to Multiple Sclerosis. *Science News* Jan. 8, 2000; Vol. 157, No. 2.

Seppa, Nathan. Chill Out: Mild Hypothermia Aids Heart Attack Recovery. *Science News* . 2002; 161(8):115.

Seppa, Nathan. Weak Appetite in Elderly Ties to Hormone. *Science News* 2001; 160:390.

Short Background of MSG. 9 June 2002.
South, James. Excitotoxins - the Ultimate Brainslayer. 23 June 2002 http:// ias-excitotoxins.htm.

Shnayerson, M. and Plotkin, M. *The Killers Within: The Deadly Rise of Drug-Resistant Bacteria.* 2002.

Spires, T., et al. Environmental Enrichment Rescues Protein Deficits. *Journal of Neuroscience.* 2004; 24(9):2270.

Spranger M., et al. Excess Glutamate in the Cerebrospinal Fluid in Bacterial Meningitis. *J. Neurol. Sci.* 1996; 143:126.

Steinman, D., Epstein, S. The Safe Shopper's Bible: A Consumer's Guide to Nontoxic Household Products.1995.Published by John Wiley & Sons.

110

Stokes, Ian. The NuTron Test. *Positive Health Magazine* 1998; 30:July.

Surtees, R., Leonard, J., and Austin, S. Association of Demyelination with Deficiency of Cerebrospinal Fluid S-adenosylmethionine in Inborn Errors of Methyl-transfer Pathway. *The Lancet* 1991; 338: 1550.

Taub, E., Ramey, S.L., DeLuca, S.C., Echols, K. Efficacy of Constrait induced (CI) Movement Therapy for Children With Cerebral Palsy. *Pediatrics*. 2004; 113(2):305.

Tamura G., et al. A Glutamine Transport Gene glnQ Is Required for Fibronectin Adherence and Virulence of Group B Streptococci. *Infection and Immunity*. 2002; 70(6):2877.

Tasker A., et al. Is Gastric Reflux a Cause of Otitis Media With Effusion in Children? *JAMA*. 2003; 289(11):1351.

Teplicky, et al. The Changes of Muscarinic , Beta adrenergic Receptors in Acetylcholinesterase Knockout Mice. Abstracts Department Physiology , Academy Sciences Czek Republic 2004.

Travers J, and E Helzner. Use of Dimercaptan Acids, Salts and Metabolites Thereof as Antiretroviral Treatment *US Patent* 1995.

Travis, John. Cancer Drugs may Thwart Huntington's. *Science News* 2001; 160(21): 332.

Travis, John. Drugs tested for Lou Gehrig's disease. *Science News* 2001; 160(23):362.

Travis, John. The Science of Secretin. *Science News.*2001;160:314.

Travis, John, Stimulating Clue hints How Lithium Works. *Science News Online* Feb. 14, 1998.

Tsakiris, S. Alanine Reverses the Inhibility Effect of Phenylalanine on Acetylchlinesterase Activity. *Z. Naturforsch*. 2002; 57c

Vaccines: The MMR Vaccine. 1 May 2002 http://vaccines-mmr.html.

Vaccine Scandal Revives Cancer Fear. *New Scientist.* 7 July 2004.

Vader, W., et al. The HLA-DQ2 Gene Dose Effect in Celiac Disease. *PNAS.* 2003;10:1073.

Vitamin K. *Life Extension Magazine.* 2000; 25 Mar. 2002 http://www.lef.org/magazine/mag2000/feb00-report.html.

Vojdani, A., et al. Antibodies to Neuron-specific Antigens in Children with Autism. *J of Neuroimmunology.* 2003;129 (1): 168.

Waly, M., et al. Activation of Methione Synthase by Insulin-like Growth Factor-1 and Dopamine. *Molecular Psychiatry.* 2004; 1-13.

Ward D., et al. Direct Mercuration of Nucleotides and Polynucleotides. *Biochemistry* 1975; 14(11):2447.

Weinstein, Y., et al. Sex Associated Differences in the Regulation of Immune Responses Controlled by the MHC of the Mouse. *J of Immunology.* 1984; 132:656.

Wells and Wilkins, Clostridia http://gsbs.utmb.edu/microbook/ch018.htm. What are Hydrolyzed Proteins. 22 June 2002 <http://msg.html>.

What Came Before DNA? *Discover.* June 2004.

Williams D. Muck Up a Leaky Gut. *Alternatives.* 2003; February:156.

Williams D. Magnetically Attractive Healing. *Alternatives.* 2004; March:65.

Woodbury, D. J., Miller, C. Nystatin induced liposome fusion: A versatile approach to ion channel reconstitution into planar bilayers. *Biophys. J.* 1990; 58:833.

Wunderlich V, and G. Sydow. Disintegration of Retroviruses by Chelating Agents. *Archives of Virology* 1982; 73:171.

Yasko A. The Role of Excitotoxins in Autistic Type Behavior. www.holistichealth.com. 2002; June 16.

Yasko A. Autism: A Twisted Tale of Virus and Thimerosal. www.holistichealth.com. 2003; May 31.

Yu, A J and Dayan, P. Acetylcholine, Norepinephrine, and Spatial Attention. Elsevier computer Science Preprint Server, 2003.

Zhu, B. COMT Mediated Methylation Metabolism of Endogenous Bioactive Catehols. *Current Drug Metabolism.* 2002; 3(3): 321.

Zhu H., et al. Cu (2+) Suppresses GABA (A) Receptor-Mediated Responses in Rat Sacral Dorsal Commissural Neurons. *Neurosignals* 2002; 11(6): 322.

Zubieta, J., et al. COMT Val 158met Genotype Affects u-Opioid Neurotransmitter Responses to a Pain Stressor. *Science.* 2003; 299(5610): 1240.

Zweiger, Gary. *Transducing the Genome.* 2001.

# Appendix

## Supplements & Descriptions

**Note**: References supporting the use of these supplements can be found at www.holistichealth.com.

**Vitamin A-** (beta carotene) This vitamin has a bit of a mixed "pedigree". Vitamin A is a fat-soluble vitamin, so it has the potential to accumulate in tissues and cause liver toxicity. Conversely, if an individual has difficulties with fat absorption, they may actually be deficient in Vitamin A. Alcohol can enhance the toxicity of Vitamin A. Elevated levels of Vitamin A are associated with an increased risk of hip fracture in women. On the other hand, Vitamin A is an antioxidant, neutralizing free radicals. There have been some studies, which suggest that high levels of Vitamin A may increase the risk of certain cancers, including breast cancer and lung cancer. However, other studies have shown Vitamin A to be useful in combating cervical cancer. This condition has been correlated with infection by the human papilloma virus. Vitamin A is often recommended for children with autism. This may stem from work in Africa, which found that high doses of Vitamin A were useful in reducing the severity of measles viral infection. Subsequent work has shown that while Vitamin A is useful to help eradicate virus if there is a Vitamin A deficiency, it can actually promote viral transmission if there is no deficiency. This may explain some of the divergent results with the use of Vitamin A. Caution should be used when considering the use of high doses of Vitamin A.

**Acidophilus-** This is a probiotic, or the natural bacteria that line your intestinal tract. It is important to repopulate your body with normal flora. Acidophilus is one of several types of probiotics. The most basic is simply acidophilus. **Allerdophilus** works in a similar fashion, but is designed for allergic individuals. **Kyodophilus** is a chewable form that works well for young children.

**Supremadophilus** is an excellent probiotic. It contains normal flora, FOS, which is basically food to help producing healthy bacteria levels for the normal bacteria grow.

**Adrenal Support-** Adrenal insufficiency occurs when the adrenals are unable to produce normal amounts of hormones, or when the body has a reduced capacity to deal with chronic stress. A professional health care practitioner who may advise the use of an Adrenal Supplement best diagnoses this condition.

**Alpha Lipoic Acid-** This helps to increase glutathione in the liver. It supplies a sulfur group to the body. It is also one of the few antioxidants that are able to work in both the water and the fat phases in the body. As a result it is able to help with oxidized cholesterol. It is often used in conjunction with other sulfur containing supplements for heavy metal detoxification when used as part of the diet to maintain healthy blood.

**Artichoke-** This works well in conjunction with **Yellow Dock** to relieve occasional constipation. It is a nice addition to a daily supplement regime, with or without the yellow dock. It will also help to maintain cholesterol levels that are already in the normal range.

**ATP-** This can be used as an alternative, or in conjunction with **NADH,** as a source of energy to help with detoxification. Your brain needs adequate stores of ATP in order to detoxify harmful substances.

**B Complex-** This will help build nerves and form acetylcholine; it should also be used in conjunction with **SAMe** supplementation. B vitamins are particularly critical for memory. They also help to make acetylcholine that has been shown to be correlated with memory issues. B vitamins help the liver, help the body to deal with stress. Stress depletes B vitamins. They are water-soluble; any excess is excreted so B's need to be supplemented on a daily basis. Excess

B's may turn urine a bright yellow- this is fine! It is important to take B vitamins as a complex, as it has been shown that taking a single B vitamin will deplete the levels of the other B vitamin's and this occurs in a dose dependent fashion. For example, a central inflammatory mediator in other neurological inflammation is homocysteine. Lack of particular B's will increase the homocysteine levels in the blood. A general B supplement should help to lower homocysteine levels.

**B12-** (methylcobolamine) This is one of the B vitamins. Unlike the other B vitamins this form of B is degraded in the stomach so most of it is destroyed when it is swallowed. The individual B12s melt in the mouth like a mint, so they can be absorbed without being degraded. They help to balance glutamate and GABA, and serve as methyl donors. They are great for energy and to fight fatigue. They have been found to help with motion sickness and to calm nervousness. There are reports to suggest that B12 helps to regenerate nerves. It is a good idea to supplement with a variety of forms of B12 simultaneously, using the cyano form, the methyl form, and the hydroxy forms of B12.

**Bacopa-** This ayurvedic herb works nicely in conjunction with **Gotu Kola**. It has been reported to help with communication between the left and right sides of the brain. Using bacopa with gotu kola has been helpful in terms of communication.

**Black cohosh-** This herb is useful to offset mild symptoms of menopause. It works well in conjunction with **Vitex** and **Dong Quai**. If that combination is not successful then the product listed as **Natural Estrogen** will often help to remedy symptoms of menopause. It is a good idea to also supplement with **Indole 3 Carbinol** when using black cohosh.

**Borage Oil-** This is an excellent source of both omega 3 and omega 6 essential fatty acids. Borage Oil works especially well to soothe dry irritated skin. Borage Oil can be taken orally as well as a topical lotion (**Shikai**). Some individuals prefer borage oil to evening primrose oil for "PMS type symptoms" or breast soreness associated with menstrual cycles, and found that it is more effective for these conditions.

**Boswellia-** It supports joint health and maintenance. It works best as part of a "trio" along with **Curcumin** and **Nettle**.

**Branched Chain Amino Acids-** This helps to protect the blood brain barrier, and to control glutamate. This supplement should not be used if a maple syrup smell is apparent in the urine.

**Broccoli-** Most of us do not eat enough broccoli, so it is nice to be able to enhance our levels with a supplement. Broccoli is a wonderful source of sulfur. The more sulfur the better, especially when it comes to neurological health.

**Buffer pH-** This supplement is best used in combination with a pH kit. This way you can determine the pH of your urine or saliva before attempting to balance your pH. This supplement when used in conjunction with a pH kit will aid in maintaining proper PH balance in the body.

**Burdock Root-** This is an especially good supplement to purify and detoxify the body in a gentle fashion. We are all exposed to so many stressors and toxins in our everyday lives. This is an easy way to try to undo some of that damage on a daily basis.

**Burpleurum-** This has been reported to be helpful in supporting the liver.

**Vitamin C-** This helps with the absorption of nutrients in the brain, thus increasing their ability to cross the blood brain barrier. Vitamin C also helps to regenerate glutathione, a critical detoxification substance that is made by the liver. The more vitamin C, the better, as long as it doesn't cause problems with loose bowels.

**Calcium-** The best calcium supplements contain calcium, magnesium, vitamin D and vitamin K. A number of practitioners are not huge supporters of the current trend toward massive doses of calcium. Based on expertise with neurological inflammation, large doses of calcium can actually be detrimental to the body. All the calcium in the world will not get to where it is needed in the body without sufficient vitamin D and vitamin K. Many people who believe they are calcium deficient are actually low in the fat-soluble vitamins D and K. As we age, our ability to break down fats and assimilate these vitamins may decrease. Taking high doses of calcium can also deplete the body's stores of magnesium. Magnesium is helpful for the heart, for blood sugar levels and for muscle cramping. Calcium supplements are available that contain vitamin D and vitamin K to help with the absorption of calcium, as well as a ratio of 750 mg of calcium to 500 mg of magnesium to help keep these mineral in balance. For those who desire a 1:1 ratio of calcium to magnesium, you can add additional 250mg magnesium. While there have been reports that calcium helps with weight loss, it has also been reported in the literature that there is an inverse relationship between osteoporosis and hormone sensitive cancers. What this study implies is that the higher the bone density, the greater the risk of beast cancer. This is another reason to use moderation with respect to calcium.

**Candex-** There have been reports of great success with the use of this supplement to help balance flora. It should be used in conjunction with a number of other supplements designed to restore a balance to the normal flora in the body.

**Carnitine-** This has been found to be helpful for the heart and for the liver. It also is useful in converting fat into energy, increasing the energy in the mitochondria that are the energy storage centers in your cells, and helping to maintain cholesterol levels that are already in the normal range.

**Carnosine + Rosemary-** Carnosine has been reported to help break down beta amyloid plaque and to limit the hexamer reaction in the body. It may also help to reduce both iron and copper in the system, thereby aiding in the balance of the copper/zinc ratio. Rosemary helps to keep the Carnosine intact so that it can do its job. Taken together, this combination works really well.

**Cascara sagrada-** This supplement is excellent for those with sluggish bowels. Cascara is reported to be non-habit forming, so it can be useful for those who are trying to break a laxative dependency. It has also been described to strengthen the colon and help promote and maintain its health. This supplement works well in conjunction with **Artichoke** and **Yellow Dock**.

**Cell Food-** A few drops of this liquid supplement can be added to a drink or a glass of water to provide a wide range of minerals, enzymes and other nutrients. Cell Food is a nice accompaniment to a detoxification program or a chelation program to ensure that you do not become depleted in minerals.

**Chamomile-** This is traditionally used as a calming herb and for help with sleep. It is actually a natural source of calcium. However, chamomile also helps to maintain healthy levels of the enzyme control MAPkinase. This is a good supplement for those who are concerned about their calcium intake, yet at the same time would like to prevent inflammation as a result of calcium.

**Cherry Extract-** This is an excellent supplement when fresh tart cherries are out of season. This supplement is exceedingly helpful for high uric acid conditions.

**Choachol-** This is a gall bladder supplement that has a simple yet effective suggested use. It has been reported to help individuals who have had their gall bladders removed. A number of individuals have had tremendous success using this supplement to counter the "dumping syndrome" often encountered after gall bladder removal.

**Choline-** This is a specific supplement that is in the B family. Choline will work to directly help to synthesize additional acetylcholine. While there is choline in the B complex, additional choline is a good idea in individuals with memory problems associated with aging.

**Chondroitin-** Many people like to take a combination of glucosamine plus chondroitin for joint support. Others prefer a separate chondroitin supplement that is formulated to be well absorbed. Many Chondroitin supplements or combination supplements are of a high molecular weight and are not easily absorbed. It is important to use low molecular weight Chondroitin. It also works well with **Glucosamine/MSM** supplements.

**Citrimax-** This contains **Chromium Picolinate** to help with blood sugar, as well as garcinia, which is an extract from citrus fruit. It has been reported to help stimulate the metabolism and aid in weight management. This supplement works well taken in conjunction with a **Green Tea** oral supplement.

**Cod Liver Oil-** This is an excellent supplement for those who want to support the liver, or those who have issues with occasional constipation. Many individuals prefer a gel cap supplement, which can be swallowed, over liquid forms of cod liver oil.

**Collagen-** This supplement is often utilized for skin health, as well as to support joint health. It is often helpful for individuals who need joint support when a glucosamine/chondroitin supplement has been unable to make a difference.

**Collinsonia-** (otherwise known as **Stone root)** This herb is helpful for strengthening the veins. Many individuals prefer this supplement to butchers broom for this purpose, as it should not create potential blood pressure issues as can occur with butcher's broom. Horse chestnut is another good supplement for vein strength. Horse chestnut is also available as a topical cream. It can be used in conjunction with collinsonia. For those with blood pressure issues the safest approach would be an oral collinsonia supplement with or without topical cream.

**Complete Vitamin and Ultra Antioxidant-** This includes vitamins, antioxidants, and minerals to lay the nutritional groundwork. It is preferable to use a complete vitamin that is specially formulated with neurological inflammation in mind. It should have no copper, no iron and limited calcium relative to magnesium. In addition to all the essential vitamins and minerals it should contain milk thistle, N-acetyl cysteine, and selenium to help the body make glutathione (a critical antioxidant made in the liver). It should also include pine bark extract (pycnogenol) to protect the glutamate receptors, and taurine to help balance glutamate and GABA.

**Colostrum-** This helps to support the immune system. Colostrum is particularly helpful for stomach and intestinal health.

**CoQ10-** This can be thought of as the "currency" that the cells of your body trade in rather than money. As a result, it is important for your cells to have adequate stores of CoQ10. This will help with energy, build new nerves and help with membrane fluidity. Based on a recent NIH study, more is better with CoQ10. CoQ10 is an important antioxidant for oxidative damage in the body, including in the fat phase, not simply the water phase in the cells. There have been reports that indicate that low levels of CoQ10 are a factor in congestive heart failure. Any individual taking statin drugs should be supplementing with CoQ10 on a daily basis.

**Cox 2 Support Mixture-** This is a combination of a number of supplements that are reported to help support fluid balance in joints. Natural joint support supplements include phellodendron, tumeric ginger, white willow, boswellia, devil's claw, green tea, bromelain, papain, protease, grape seed, rosemary, quercetin and polygonum.

**Cranberry-** This supplement has a reputation for being helpful for urinary tract health. There is literature to support its ability to maintain flora balance. Cranberry works well in conjunction with a number of other supplements that may have antimicrobial properties. One group that works extremely well together is **Oregon grape, Neem, Myrrh, Golden Seal, Cranberry, and Oregamax, +/- Uva Ursi.**

**Curbita-** This is an extract from pumpkin. There are reports to suggest that pumpkin extract helps to strengthen the bladder muscles.

**Curcumin-** This is a truly excellent supplement. It is a natural promoter of joint/cartilage health, which is helpful to those looking for joint support. It also works nicely as part of a "trio" along with **Boswellia** and **Nettle**. Curcumin has also been reported to be helpful in promoting colon and skin health. It serves as a methyl donor.

**Vitamin D-** This can be taken in winter or in cloudy regions to supplement the vitamin D in the General Vitamin. Adequate levels of vitamin D are important to immune health. A correlation has been found between areas of the country with reduced sun exposure and healthy levels of Vitamin D.

**Dandelion Leaf-** This supplement taken several times daily is very helpful to support the kidneys and bladder. It works nicely in combination with taurine and SAMe with a B complex for kidney health.

**Dandelion Root-** While dandelion leaf is lovely for the kidneys, dandelion root helps to support the liver. The liver is one of the most important organs in the body. It is responsible for detoxification in the body, and the liver synthesizes glutathione, which is critical for detoxification and immune support. Supporting the liver is therefore of utmost importance. Dandelion root works well with **Milk Thistle** for liver support.

**DHEA-** For years this supplement was touted as the fountain of youth, helping to offset aging. It is true that as we age, our DHEA levels decline along with estrogen or testosterone. It has also been reported to be helpful in a variety of immune boosting mechanisms. DHEA can be of use when an individual has low levels of DHEA. However, it is not wise to supplement with DHEA unless you have confirmed the fact that your levels are low and in need of supplementation. Taking a supplement that can increase hormone levels is a double-edged sword. If you need it then it may be extremely helpful to supplement. If you do not need it, you may run the risk of increasing hormone levels to a point where you could cause abnormal growth in your body.

**Digestive Enzymes-** There are two types of digestive enzymes that work especially well when used together, **Super Digestive Enzymes** and **Ultra Dairy**. This pair of enzymes help with bloating, the digestion of fats, support the pancreas, help with minor blood sugar issues, and may help with acid neutralization. It is a good idea to take one of each with every meal.

**DMG (dimethyl glycine)-** The glycine can stimulate the glutamate activity when glutamate is still in excess. As the glutamate is more under control, then the DMG will work well in conjunction with GABA. DMG is also a very good methyl donor. Methylation is important for autism. DMG can also be helpful for neurological health.

**Dong Quai-** This supplement is useful to offset symptoms of menopause. It works well in conjunction with vitex and black cohosh. If that combination is not successful then the product listed as Natural Estrogen will often help. As with black cohosh, this supplement may be useful in stimulating language. It is best used in conjunction with indole 3 carbinol.

**Dopa 400-** This natural source of dopa is derived from Mucuna pruriens, or the Velvet Bean. This supplement is helpful for individuals who want to supplement their natural dopamine levels. Imbalances in dopamine levels are known to be a problem in Parkinson's disease. Dopamine imbalances have also been implicated in autism, addictive behaviors and in ADD.

**Vitamin E-** This is a well-known supplement taken as an antioxidant to help with heart health, prostate health, and perhaps most importantly to regenerate glutathione. Vitamin E is part of a family of supplements known as tocopherols. Vitamin E that is a combination of mixed tocopherols has been reported to be more effective than individual vitamin E supplements.

**Echinacea-** This is a classic herb that is used to support the immune system. It is most effective if used as a trio, in conjunction with **Elderberry** and **Goldenseal**. Echinacea should not be used as a daily supplement. Rather, it should only be used when needed. Individuals with allergies should be cautious in their use of this herb; individuals with autoimmune conditions should avoid the use of Echinacea.

**EDTA-** This supplement works extremely well in chelating metals without the side effects seen with other chelating agents. There is also extensive literature available concerning the use of EDTA to help support the heart.

**EFA (essential fatty acids) + Neuromins-** This combination provides a ideal ratio of omega 3/6/9.

**Elderberry-** This herb is excellent for supporting the gut.

**Fenugreek-** This supplement will help heal the gut, increase milk production for breast-feeding and help balance sugar levels when used as part of the diet.

**Feverfew-** This herb helps in the prevention of migraine headaches.

**Fish Oil-** Fish oil is helpful for maintaining cholesterol levels that are already in the normal range.

**Folic Acid-** While folic acid is generally included in most B complexes, it is worth considering additional supplementation of this particular B vitamin. Folic acid helps to reduce homocysteine. High levels of homocysteine do not promote heart health. Folic acid is important in helping to prevent neural tube defects. It is also involved in the important methylation pathways in the body. In some cases, alternative sources of folic acid are necessary due to blocks in the pathway of folate metabolism. In these cases the use of **FolaPro (5 methyl folate)**, and or **Folinic Acid** should be considered.

**GABA-** This is a calming neurotransmitter in the body that helps to balance glutamate. It should be useful to help decrease stress, and increase speech, eye contact, and social interactions. GABA comes in several forms and it will be a bit of trial and error to determine which is best. **GABA Calm** seems to work well for many individuals during the day; it melts in the mouth like a lozenge. For those who do not like the taste or prefer to swallow a pill, **GABA** is also available as a supplement to be swallowed. **ZEN** (GABA and Theanine) is nice to take later in the evening as it helps with sleep and stress. 127

**Garlic-** This has the potential to do many wonderful things: help control cholesterol, help the liver, maintain cholesterol levels that are already in the normal range and participate in sulfur reactions in body.

**Ginkgo-** This has been reported to increase blood flow to the brain and to protect from damage due to nitric oxide. It may also help to slow the breakdown of dopamine as it has been reported to act as

126

an MAO-B inhibitor. Ginkgo should be used with caution in individuals with blood pressure issues.

**Glucosamine/MSM-** Many people like to take a combination of glucosamine chondroitin for joint support. Others prefer a separate **chondroitin** supplement that is formulated to be well absorbed. Many **chondroitin** supplements or combination supplements are of a high molecular weight and are not easily absorbed.

**Glucose support-** There are a number of nutritional supplements and herbs that can be used as part of the diet to help maintain healthy blood sugar levels. Combinations are available that include many of the herbs that may help, such as Vitamin E, magnesium, zinc, manganese, chromium, lagerstroemia speciosa, bitter melon, gymnema sylvestre, vanadyl sulfate, Jerusalem artichoke, fenugreek, milk thistle, ginkgo biloba, bilberry, alpha lipoic acid, citric bioflavonoids.

**Glutathione-** This is one of the most important supplements made by the body. It is helpful in programs designed to promote immune and neurological health. There are also reports that suggest that glutathione is useful for cystic fibrosis. If glutathione is not specially formulated it degrades in the stomach if it is swallowed.

**Goldenseal-** This works well in conjunction with a number of other supplements that may have antimicrobial properties. One group that works extremely well together is **Oregon Grape, Neem, Myrrh, Goldenseal, Cranberry, and Oregamax, +/- Uva Ursi.**

**Gotu Kola-** This ayurvedic herb is excellent in conjunction with **Bacopa**. It has been reported to help with communication between the left and right sides of the brain. Using bacopa with gotu kola has been helpful with communication.

**Grape Seed Extract-** This is reported to help to control glutamate by protecting the glutamate receptors and to support nerve health in the brain. It works well in conjunction with pycnogenol.

**Green Tea-** There are so many good things about green tea as a supplement. It has been described as helpful in everything from immune health, skin health, to increasing the metabolism for weight management.

**Guarana-** This nutritional supplement has many times the level of caffeine found in coffee. Caffeine is not always a negative. It may be helpful for many individuals who need extra pick-up. There is also information to suggest that caffeine can help with apoptosis.

**Guggulipid-Ayur-** This is useful in supporting the thyroid, for adolescent non-cystic acne, and to support the immune system.

**Gymnema-Ayur-** This is an ayurvedic herb that helps to support the pancreas health, and can be used as part of the diet to help maintain blood sugar levels. If used on a regular basis this works well for children who become "hyper" after ingesting sugar.

**Hawthorn-** This supplement is often thought of as a general heart tonic for overall heart wellness. It is a good idea to supplement with this herb for optimal heart health. This supplement works nicely in combination with **CoQ10.**

**Helix-** This nutrient provides breast health support.

**Hops-** There is literature that supports the use of hops to help balance hormone levels. It has been reported to help to convert testosterone to estrogen. This may be helpful in hormonal imbalances and in adolescent non-cystic acne. It would be wise to take **Indole 3 Carbinol** and or **Broccoli** in conjunction with hops to help keep the estrogen of the healthier type.

**Horse chestnut-** This is often used to support weak veins. It works nicely when used in conjunction with **Collinsonia**.

**Horsetail grass-** This is reportedly a rich source of silica. Horsetail grass can be helpful in aiding in bone health development. It may also be useful in helping to detoxify aluminum from the body.

**Indole 3 Carbinol-** This supplement has been described to help keep estrogen as the "healthy" type in the body. This can be taken as a daily supplement and is helpful for breast health.

**Inositol and IP6-** Inositol has been reported to be useful for helping to control obsessive behaviors. Inositol is also useful for supplementation to the muscles. Some practitioners prefer IP6 to standard inositol.

**Juniper Berry-** This has been described as being useful for urinary tract health. It is a reasonably strong supplement so it is not generally suggested for everyday use. A potentially more important use of Juniper Berry may be in breast health.

**Vitamin K-** Since glycosylation occurs as a result of sugar hooking onto protein in an incorrect fashion, supplements that help with sugar regulation should also help to decrease glycosylation. Vitamin K helps to control sugar. It also helps with bleeding and bruising. Vitamin K is a fat-soluble vitamin but it is not stored in the body like the other fat-soluble vitamins. Vitamin K needs to be made by the body or taken as a supplement on a daily, or every other day, basis. Some studies show that vitamin K is more powerful than vitamin E and coenzyme Q10 for scavenging free radicals and in other studies vitamin K by itself completely protected the liver from free radicals. Vitamin E and glutathione protect vitamin K's antioxidant effect.

**Kelp-** This is a rich source of iodine. Many years ago the purpose behind putting iodine in salt was precisely to help prevent iodine deficiency. In today's society, where many of us restrict our salt intake, we may be lacking in iodine. Kelp can be used as another means of replacing iodine rather than table salt. Sufficient iodine is important for the proper functioning of the thyroid gland.

**Lactoferrin-** This is an all-natural extract from milk.

**Liv-Ora-** This whole organ extract support for the liver.

**Lobelia-** This is a powerful and potentially dangerous supplement. It can be helpful for breaking addictive behaviors including cigarette smoking. The best idea is to use minimal quantities of this supplement, only for as long as is necessary.

**Lutein Plus-** This supplement is a lovely combination of several supplements that have been reported to be helpful in supporting eye health. It includes lutein, zeaxanithin, bilberry, and a bit of vitamin E.

**Lycopene-** There are a number of studies to suggest that lycopene is helpful for the prostate and for cancer prevention.

**Lysine-** This amino acid has been reported to help with viral infections.

**Magnesium-** This helps to block the flow of calcium into the neurons. Some individuals find that they have loose stools from too much magnesium. Conversely, magnesium is useful for constipation. Magnesium is helpful for the heart, for blood sugar levels, PMS, for muscle cramping and for lung health. There is some concern about the excessive amounts of calcium that many individuals are ingesting. It may be causing magnesium deficiencies, which may be even more dangerous.

**Malic acid-** The use of malic acid with magnesium is a good idea for individuals in need of immune supprot. It is also helpful in chelating aluminum.

**Marshmallow-** This supplement can be used to help soothe inflamed areas. It works well for everything from throat health to urinary tract health. It works best as an addition to other more targeted supplement.

**Mastica gum-** Mastica gum can be helpful for individuals looking for skin, stomach, gastric and intestinal health support.

**Melatonin-** This supplement is useful for aiding in sleep. Melatonin is also reported to be a powerful antioxidant in the brain. Several types of melatonin are available - **immediate release** is suggested for those who occasionally have trouble falling asleep. **Time release** is suggested for those who can fall asleep, but wake up during the night and can't get back to sleep. And a combination product, **Natural Sleep** is suggested for those who occasionally have trouble both falling asleep and staying asleep.

**Melissa-** This herb has been suggested to help relieve cold sores.

**Milk Thistle-** The liver is a central organ that is involved in contributing to neurological health. There is milk thistle in some general vitamins; however, in this case, more is better. Milk Thistle helps to balance liver enzyme levels, improves glutathione levels, builds new nerves and helps maintain liver health.

**Minerals-** There are several types of mineral supplementation, **Bio Nativus** liquid trace mineral drops that can be put in drinking water, and an **Ultra Mineral** supplement that can be swallowed.

**Mistletoe-** There have been reports in the literature that suggests the use of mistletoe may be helpful in immune health. It is best used as part of a more comprehensive program that includes a number of supplements to achieve optimal results.

**Moducare-** This supplement has been reported to help with viral infections.

**Mycoceutics (mushrooms + beta glucan)-** There are a number of mushroom supplements on the market. Products that have a wonderful combination of a variety of mushrooms, in addition to beta-glucan, seem to work best. This supplement should be used as part of a more complete program to support the immune system.

**Myrrh-** This works well in conjunction with a number of other supplements that may have antimicrobial properties. One group that works extremely well together is **Oregon Grape, Neem, Myrrh, Golden Seal, Cranberry, Oregamax +/- Uva Ursi.** Myrrh has also been reported to be helpful for low platelet levels. 1

**N-acetyl-cysteine-** This helps the liver to make glutathione. NAC is particularly good for the lungs and has been found to be useful for respiratory health and when used as part of the diet to help maintain healthy blood sugar levels. It should always be taken with Vitamin C.

**NADH-** This is important in energy production, particularly in the Krebs cycle. It is often useful to supplement with NADH if you are using glutathione as it helps to regenerate the glutathione to the reduced form without depleting the body's stores of NADH. This supplement is useful for neurological health.

**Natural Estrogen-** This supplement will often help to remedy symptoms of menopause. It works well in conjunction with topical **progesterone cream**.

**Neem-** This works well in conjunction with a number of other supplements that may have antimicrobial properties. One group that works extremely well together is **Oregon Grape, Neem, Myrrh, Goldenseal, and Cranberry, Oregamax +/- Uva Ursi.**

**Nettle-** This works nicely to help maintain joint fluid balance, promote joint health and skin health. It works best as part of a "trio" along with **curcumin** and **boswellia**. Nettle is also a good source of boron, which is excellent for the bones.

**Neuromins-** This is a wonderful source of omega 3 fatty acids. It is a good idea to use Neuromins, or DHA in conjunction with a complete EFA for the optimal balance of omega 3, 6, 9 fatty acids.

**No-Phenol-** This supplement is designed to help individuals who have difficulty ingesting substances that contain phenol molecules.

**Ora-Triplex-** A whole organ support for the immune system, to include the spleen, liver, and thymus extracts.

**Oregamax-** This works well in conjunction with a number of other supplements that may have antimicrobial properties. One group that works extremely well together is **Oregon Grape, Neem, Myrrh, Goldenseal, and Cranberry, Oregamax +/- Uva Ursi.**

**Oregon Grape-** This works well in conjunction with a number of other supplements that may have antimicrobial properties. One group that works extremely well together is **Oregon Grape, Neem, Myrrh, Goldenseal, Cranberry, Oregamax +/- Uva Ursi.**

**Oxydrene-** According to the available literature this supplement should be useful in increasing oxygenation in the body. In addition to adequate ATP, your brain needs sufficient oxygenation to protect itself and to detoxify harmful substances. Oxydrene has been found to have positive effects on neurological inflammation.

**PABA (Para Amino Benzoic Acid)-** While this B vitamin is included in general B complexes it is worth considering additional supplementation of PABA in individuals who want additional thyroid support.

**Pancreas-Ora-** A whole organ extract support for the pancreas.

**Pantothenic Acid-** While this B vitamin is included in general B complexes it is worth considering additional supplementation of Pantothenic Acid to help maintain cholesterol levels already within the normal range.

**Papaya-** This is a very tasty chewable supplement that can help with digestion. Papaya is a rich source of enzymes that have been described to be useful for skin as well as for digestion.

**Paradex-** This is the best combination of supplements that have been found to help control parasites.

**Parsley-** This herb has been described to have gentle diuretic and laxative properties.

**Pau d Arco-** This works best as part of a more complete program to support the immune system.

**Petadolex-** This is an excellent source of butterbur. There are a number of articles describing the use of **butterbur** to help alleviate migraine headaches and severe allergies.

**Phaseolamin-** This is an extract from the white kidney bean that has been reported to help decrease fat absorption. This is a nice supplement to use in conjunction with an overall weight management program.

**Phosphatidyl serine-** This increases acetylcholine as well as decreases stress and helps with membrane fluidity that may be compromised due to oxidized cholesterol. This is a membrane component that helps to coat nerves. It functions to protect nerves in a similar fashion to the way the rubber or plastic coating insulates electric wiring. A good source of phosphatidyl serine, phosphatidyl choline and phosphatidyl inositol.

**Placenta-Ora-** A whole organ extract support that contains placental extracts.

**Policosanol-** This helps to maintain cholesterol levels that are already in the normal range and to increase membrane fluidity.

**Primal Defense-** This supplement is a nice accompaniment to a detoxification program or a chelation program to ensure that you do not become depleted in a variety of nutrients and provides a full spectrum of organisms to promote and then maintain an optimal bowel flora. It works far better with appropriate fiber support such as **Beyond Fiber**.

**Progesterone Cream-** This topical cream can be used to help balance hormone levels.

**Psyllium Husk-** This is often used by individuals with bowel or constipation issues. Another excellent supplement combination for constipation is artichoke, yellow dock, and +/- cascara sagrada as needed. However, psyllium husk is a traditional standby that will help.

**Pycnogenol-** This can be used to help to control glutamate by protecting the glutamate receptors, as well as to help revitalize nerves. Pycnogenol is also reported to help strengthen veins.

**Quercetin-** This may help to prevent histamine release. Quercetin helps to retain the levels of carnosine in the body. Quercetin can also be useful for promoting eye health. Quercetin is also reported to help lower uric acid levels, and be helpful for prostate health.

**Relaxation-** This supplement is a combination of a number of calming and relaxing herbs to help with stress reduction or tension, which includes Theanine, oat, magnolia, chamomile, lemon balm, valerian, scullcap, hops, passionflower, magnesium, and B-6. This combination may help to increase the number of GABA receptors.
**Rosemary-** This herb is reported to be helpful for memory, and to help increase glutathione levels. Rosemary also helps to keep the **Carnosine** intact so that it can function properly. This combination works really well when taken together.

**Rhubarb-** This herb is reported to be useful in helping to stem bleeding problems. There is also literature that supports its use to help aid in occasional constipation without causing diarrhea.

**SAMe (s-adenosyl methionine)-** This is wonderful for the liver. SAMe is also a methyl donor and a sulfur donor for the following reactions in the body. The sulfur donating function is important for detoxification. SAMe is also useful to help the body get rid of excess ammonia. Because SAMe can increase serotonin levels, it can help to elevate the mood. High doses of SAMe are also reported to be highly effective for joint support. A complete B complex should be taken with each SAMe.

**Saw Palmetto-** This supplement should be considered as a part of a daily health regime for males.

**Saw Palmetto Plus Pygeum-** This supplement is similar to the standard saw palmetto with a few additional ingredients that may benefit older men.

**Selenium-** This is an important mineral helping to recycle the glutathione in your body. Selenium can be toxic in high doses, so this is not a case of more is better.

**Serraflazyme-** This supplement is reported to help break down excess mucous. It can be particularly helpful for those who suffer from chronic mucous build up, or during the winter months when congestion can be an issue.

**SerenAid-** This is often used as a digestive aid for individuals on a GFCF diet, those unable to digest gluten and casein. SerenAid is also another name for DPP-IV, which is a soluble peptidase involved in immune regulation. This enzyme may also be helpful in supporting the immune system. There is a report in the literature that DDP-IV may be helpful in melanoma.

**Slippery Elm-** This supplement works well for irritated areas.

**Soy Isoflavone-** There has been a great deal of literature to support the use of soy supplements. Supplementation with soy is best used in moderation.

**Spirulina-** The use of this blue/green algae works nicely in conjunction with MGN3 or IP6. There are articles to suggest that Spirulina helps to move natural killer cells from the blood stream into the tissues. Combining supplements that are described to help increase natural killer cell activity, with a supplement to move these immune surveillance cells into the tissues, would be using these supplements to their best advantage.

**St. Johns Wort-** This supplement is a classic in terms of its use for mood, stress and other emotional issues. Other supplements that may work better for emotional conditions are **SAMe** with a **B complex** or one of the **GABA** supplements.

**Taurine-** This is an amino acid that is not considered as an essential amino acid in the body. However, individuals who do not eat a lot of red meat are deficient in taurine. Taurine may be useful to the liver by increasing bile output. This helps in the digestion and assimilation of fats and fat-soluble vitamins. Taurine is very useful in controlling imbalances in glutamate and GABA. It may be that taurine is helpful in curtailing the rapid outpouring of taurine is reported to be useful in promoting kidney health maintaining blood pressure levels that are already with in the normal range and when used as part of the diet to maintain healthy blood sugar levels.

**Theanine-** This is the calming component from green tea. It mimics glutamate and can help protect against excessive glutamate levels.

**Thyroid/L-tyrosine-** This supplement helps to support the thyroid. This particular combination supplement seems to work better than plain l-tyrosine supplements.

**Tonalin (Conjugated Linoleic Acid)-** This supplement is often used in conjunction with a weight management program. CLA has been reported to help the body to burn fat.

**Transfer Factor-** This supplement is excellent for helping to support the immune system.

**Trehalose-** This is a natural sugar that has been found to decrease the formation of glutamate aggregates.

**Uva Ursi-** This works well in conjunction with a number of other supplements that may help healthy microbial support. One group that works extremely well together is **Oregon Grape, Neem, Myrrh, Golden Seal, Cranberry, and Oregamax, +/- Uva Ursi.** It is best to use Uva Ursi for two to three weeks and then discontinue it for two to three weeks.

**Vinpocetine-** This helps to increase circulation to the brain and to remove excess calcium from the brain. It can also act to inhibit microtubule formation and may therefore be useful in triggering apoptosis or programmed cell death (a natural pruning process in cells to eliminate damaged cells).

**Vital Yew-** This product is available as a supplement, which can be taken orally, and as a topical cream.

**Vitex-** This helps to balance the levels of estrogen and progesterone. Vitex is useful to offset symptoms of menopause, as well as to offset symptoms of PMS. For symptoms of menopause it works well in conjunction with black cohosh and dong quai. If that combination is not successful then the product listed as **Natural Estrogen** will often help to remedy more severe symptoms.

**Yellow Dock-** An excellent combination to relieve constipation is **Artichoke** in conjunction with **Yellow Dock**. **Yellow Dock** is a nice addition to a daily supplement regime, with or without the **Artichoke**.

**Zinc-** This helps to block the flow of calcium into the neurons. Zinc works well for people who cannot tolerate magnesium. However, zinc is a double-edged sword; too much zinc will cause glutamate release. It is best to keep zinc at 25-40 mg per day.

# Excitotoxin Free Diet

It is virtually impossible to completely eliminate glutamate and aspartate from your diet, nor would you want to. Stimulatory activity from the glutamate receptor is important for neurotransmission. What we want to avoid is excessive stimulation of this neurotransmitter. One way to think about excitotoxins is to imagine an empty glass Pyrex measuring cup. Understand that the cup gets filled up over the course of a day or a lifetime with glutamate. The point at which the cup is overflowing represents when you are already seeing obvious signs of neurological damage. The less that you put into the cup each day, the less likely it is to overflow. The goal of this section is to give you a good sense of the sources of glutamate and aspartate so that you can make informed choices in terms of "filling your cup". It would be extremely difficult to follow a completely excitotoxin free diet "to the letter". The information presented here can be used to serve as a guideline for trying to limit the intake of excitotoxins in addition to following a gluten free/casein free diet. The idea is to keep excitotoxins to a minimum; you will never avoid them completely.

# Sources of Excitotoxins

monosodium glutamate
nutrasweet / aspartame
malted barely flour
glutamate
hydrolyzed protein
malt extract
natural flavor(s)
hydrolyzed vegetable protein
malt flavoring(s)
natural flavoring(s)
hydrolyzed plant protein
malted barley / barley malt
maltodextrin

140

hydrolyzed oat flour
malted anything
carrageenan
hydrolyze anything
textured protein
gelatin
sodium caseinate
guar gum
spice(s)
calcium caseinate
soy extract
seasoning(s)
caseinate
soy protein
seasoned salt
disodium guanylate
soy protein concentrate
dough conditioner(s)
disodium inosinate
soy protein isolate
yeast extract
disodium caseinate
soy sauce
autolyzed yeast
chicken/pork/beef "flavoring"whey protein
autolyzed yeast extract
chicken/pork/beef "base" whey protein isolate
autolyzed anything
bouillon
whey protein concentrate
broth
vegetable gum
kombu extract
stock
plant protein extract    l-cysteine
soup base
smoke flavoring(s)
ajinomoto

# Sources of MSG

## Definite Sources of MSG
- Hydrolyzed Protein
- Hydrolyzed Oat Flour
- Sodium Caseinate or Calcium Caseinate
- Autolyzed Yeast or Yeast Extract
- Gelatin
- Glutamic Acid
- Monosodium Glutamate

## Possible Sources of MSG
- Textured Protein
- Carrageenan or Vegetable Gum
- Seasonings or Spices
- Flavorings or Natural Flavorings
- Chicken, Beef, Pork, Smoke Flavorings
- Bouillon, Broth or Stock
- Barley Malt, Malt Extract, Malt Flavoring
- Whey Protein, Whey Protein Isolate or Concentrate
- Soy Protein, Soy Protein Isolate or Concentrate
- Soy Sauce or Extract

## Other Sources of MSG
- MSG is found in most food prepared by major fast-food chains.
- Binders and fillers for medications, nutrients, and supplements, both prescription and non-prescription, and some fluids administered intravenously in hospitals, may contain MSG.
- According to the manufacturer, Varivax-Merck chicken pox vacinne (Varicella Virus Live) contains L-monosodium glutamate and hydrolyzed gelatin, both of which contain processed free glutamic acid (MSG).
- MSG is used as a plant "growth enhancer" (AuxiGro) that is sprayed on growing crops. AuxiGro Plant Metabolic Primer contains 29.2% by weight, pharmaceutical grade, L-glutamic acid.
- The most common sources of MSG: molasses, sugar beet & cane.
- MSG and Aspartame (NutraSweet) are found in everything from soups, sauces, and juice to frozen entrees, candy, cigarettes, and anything with seasonings (e.g., potato chips, meat, ice cream).

**The following foods have enough MSG/Glutamate content to cause a reaction in individuals sensitive to it or contain some amount of Glutamate and should be avoided. Remember - ALWAYS read labels. Product contents can change at any time at the company's discretion.**

Doritos
Pringles
KFC fried chicken
Boar's Head cold cuts/hot dogs
Progresso Soups
Lipton Soups/Sauces
Gravy Master
Planter's salted peanuts
Sausages/Processed meats/Cold cuts
Processed cheese spread
Molasses
Supermarket turkey & chicken (injected)
Restaurant gravy from food service cans
Ramen noodles
Boullion (any kind)
Instant soup mixes/Stocks
Many salad dressings/Croutons
Most salty, powdered dry food mixes
Flavored potato chips
Restaurant soups made from food service soup base
Gelatin
Soy sauce
Worcestershire sauce
Kombu extract
Dry milk or whey powder
Dough conditioners
Body builder protein mixes
Parmesan cheese
Fresh produce sprayed with Auxigro in the field
Some spices

Skim, 1%, 2%, non-fat, or dry milk
Whipped cream topping substitutes
Non-dairy creamers
Chocolates/Candy bars
Low-fat/Diet Foods
Cereals
Baked goods from bakeries
Frostings and fillings
Catsup
Mayonnaise
Chili sauce
Mustards
Pickles
Bottled spaghetti sauce
Citric acid (when processed from corn)
Canned and smoked tuna, oysters, clams
Barbeque sauce
Canned, frozen, or dry entrees and potpies
Fresh and frozen pizza
Flavored teas, sodas
Seasoned anything
Some peanut butters
Some bagged salads and vegetables
Tomato sauce/Stewed tomatoes
Egg substitutes
Flour
Canned refried beans
Tofu and other fermented soy products
Table salts
Anything with corn syrup added
Anything with milk solids
Anything fermented
Anything vitamin enriched
Anything protein fortified
Anything enzyme modified
Anything ultra-pasteurized

144

Caramel flavoring/coloring
Pectin
Cornstarch
Flowing agents
Xanthan gum/other "gums"
L-cysteine

## High Protein Diets

All proteins contain glutamate, aspartate, and cysteine (and phenylalanine), so it is best to eat a low/moderate amount of protein, rather than a high protein diet. If you have been advised to follow the PKU (phenylalanine free) Diet, avoid or severely limit all protein-rich foods. PKU diets are designed to eliminate phenylalanine, which is a phenolic amino acid; it would be useful for phenol sensitive individuals to limit intake of phenylalanine.

Frequently, people who display Autistic type behaviors are placed on high protein diets. Because high levels of glutamate and aspartate are found naturally in protein rich foods, and excess amounts can create a wide range of bodily damage, high protein diets are not recommended for this population. The breakdown of protein also generates ammonia. Many autistic children already have issues with elevated ammonia. This is another reason to avoid high protein diets in this population.

In addition to neurological damage due to excitotoxins, high protein diets force the body into a state of cannibalism, called *Metabolic acidosis*, where blood levels become so acidic that the body starts feeding on muscle tissue for nutrients.

## Vitamin K
Because Vitamin K is enzymatically involved with glutamate and sugar metabolism, it is important for people with autistic type behavior to consume foods high in this vitamin.  Below is a list of Vitamin K rich foods:

|  |  |
| --- | --- |
| Broccoli | 200 mcg |
| Spinach | 106 mcg |
| Avocado | 80.4 mcg |
| Turnip greens | 66.8 mcg |
| Lettuce | 55.9 mcg |
| Cabbage | 48.3 mcg |
| Pistachio nuts | 42.6 mcg |
| Watercress | 40.4 mcg |
| Soybean oil | 26.2 mcg |
| Snap beans | 24.6 mcg |
| Plums | 18.8 mcg |
| Canola oil | 19.7 mcg |
| Kiwi fruit | 19.0 mcg |
| Green peas | 17.5 mcg |
| Miso | 14.4 mcg |
| Carrots | 13.3 mcg |
| Sweet peppers | 8.08 mcg |
| Potatoes | 8.10 mcg |
| Tomatoes | 7.38 mcg |
| Celery | 6.84 mcg |
| Peanut butter | 7.20 mcg |
| Olive oil | 6.62 mcg |
| Cauliflower | 5.89 mcg |
| Cucumbers | 5.72 mcg |

## Sulfur

Sulfur is necessary for the metabolism of sulfur-related proteins in the body. If sulfur is deficient, an excess of nitric oxide can result, leading to excitotoxin damage. Foods high in sulfur are listed below:

Red hot peppers
Fish
Meat
Legumes
Nuts
Eggs
Cabbage
Brussel sprouts
Dried beans
Onions
Garlic
Watercress
Horseradish
Radish
Arugula
Mustard leaves
Mustard/radish flowers

Molybdenum helps the body to process sulfur properly. If molybdenum levels are too low, then supplementation should be considered.

# About the Authors

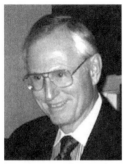

**Garry F. Gordon** MD, DO, MD (H), received his Doctor of Osteopathy in 1958 from the Chicago College of Osteopathy in Illinois. He received his honorary MD degree from the University of California Irvine in 1962 and completed his Radiology Residency from Mt. Zion in San Francisco, California in 1964. For many years, he was the Medical Director of Mineral Lab in Hayward, California, a leading laboratory for trace mineral analysis worldwide with offices in Boston, Amsterdam, and Tokyo.

Dr. Gordon is on the Board of Homeopathic Medical Examiners for Arizona and is Co-Founder of the American College for Advancement in Medicine (ACAM). He is Founder/President of the International College of Advanced Longevity (ICALM) and Board Member of International Oxidative Medicine Association (IOMA). He is also a member of the Scientific Advisory Committee for The National Foundation for Alternative Medicine.

With Morton Walker, DPM, Dr. Gordon co-authored *The Chelation Answer*. In addition, he was the instructor and examiner for all chelation physicians. Currently he is an advisor to the American Board of Chelation Therapy and responsible for Peer Review for Chelation Therapy in the State of Arizona.

As an internationally recognized expert on chelation therapy, Dr. Gordon is now attempting to establish standards for the proper use of oral and intravenous chelation therapy as an adjunct therapy for all diseases. He lectures extensively on *The End Of Bypass Surgery Is In Sight* and *The Future of Chelation*.

Currently, Dr. Gordon is President of Gordon Research Institute and a full-time consultant for Longevity Plus, a nutritional supplement company located in Payson, Arizona. He is responsible for the design of the majority of their supplements, which are widely used by alternative health practitioners around the world.

**Amy S. Yasko** Ph.D., ND, NHD, AMD, HHP, FAAIM, has extensive expertise in biochemistry, molecular biology, and biotechnology. She also has research and clinical experience in both allopathic and alternative medicine. The common thread that winds through these fields is her work with RNA.

As co-founder and owner of a successful biotechnology company, she is recognized as an expert in the field of DNA/RNA based diagnostics and therapeutics and has been a consultant to the medical and research community for eighteen years. More than twenty years ago she began isolating single copy RNA messages from transformed cells at Strong Memorial Hospital Cancer Center. Later, while at Yale Medical Center, she worked to enhance the expression of specific eukaryotic RNAs from yeast.

During her tenure at St. Vincent's Hospital in NYC, Dr. Yasko developed custom diets and used nutritional supplements to improve the cure rates of Hodgkin's disease patients. She worked with Dr. Lawrence to isolate some of the first clinical samples of Transfer Factor for use in these patients. She then went on to conduct molecular research on Transfer Factor in Dr. Fudenburg's Immunology Dept. at the Medical University of South Carolina.

Dr. Yasko was also a member of the Dept. of Pediatrics and Infectious Diseases at Strong Memorial Hospital and worked to develop safer *Haemophilus influenza* vaccines. She has also spent years studying the relationship between energy transport and

150

modes of antibiotic resistance by bacteria and has written articles and chapters in books on the subject.

Five years ago, Dr. Yasko established an alternative healthcare practice specializing in chronic inflammation, immunological and neurological disorders. To date, she has had considerable success in halting and in most cases reversing the effects of such debilitating diseases from which her clients suffer, such as ALS, MS, Parkinson's disease, Alzheimer's disease, SLE, Myasthenia gravis and autism. Most recently her primary focus has been to construct a program to help to reverse autism.

Dr. Yasko graduated cum laude with a BS in Chemistry and Fine Arts from Colgate University. She then completed her medical education at Albany Medical College and received a Doctorate in Microbiology, Immunology, and Infectious Diseases with an award for outstanding academic excellence, graduating summa cum laude. She was the first woman in that department to receive a Doctorate in this field. Dr. Yasko continued her education to graduate with high honors from the Clayton College of Natural Health, receiving two additional degrees, a Doctor of Naturopathy and a Doctor of Natural Health. She is licensed as a Naturopathic Physician and board certified as an Alternative Medical Doctor, a Holistic Health Practitioner and is a Fellow of the American Association of Integrative Medicine. Dr. Yasko is a member of the scientific advisory board for NFAM (National Foundation of Alternative Medicine). It was as a member of this board that Dr. Yasko had the opportunity to meet Dr. Garry Gordon, another NFAM board member. Dr. Gordon and Dr. Yasko's mutual interest in the use of RNA as nutritional supplements has led to a number of collaborative efforts including this book on autism.

Did you miss the exciting conference introducing this book?  Well it's all right because DVDs are now available!  These videos expand on the information contained in this book and will take you to the next level of learning about autism.

Gordon Research Institute presented this material at the Boston 2004 conference "New Dimensions In Medicine & Health--Answers on Autism", featuring Dr. Amy Yasko, Dr. Garry F. Gordon, Dr. Robert Nash and parent Robert Claeys.  This conference discussed the entire protocol found in this book in depth. You will be able to listen to the interaction between doctors and parents, answering questions from metal detoxification to nerve re-myelination.

These recordings are available through Holistic Health Consultants, L.L.C (www.holisticheal.com) and Longevity Plus-RNA, L.L.C (www.longevityplus-rna.com  / (877) 762-3663).

AUTISM ANSWER.COM

→ Nerve Inflam → Heavy Metals

Chloride blocks sulfur

NADH keeps GSH reduced

Brain energy: Ginko, NADH, Co Q(10),
Ribose, Carnitine, Vinpocetine

Heavy metals trigger ↑ Glutamate tox.

Acetyl-L-Carnitine heals liver

B6 alone "stimmy", use B Co